SAFETY FOR YOUNG CHILDREN

by Cindy Barden

illustrated by Janet Skiles and Kathryn Marlin

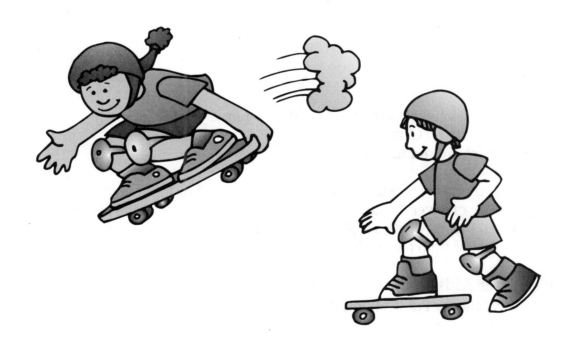

Fearon Teacher Aids
A Division of Frank Schaffer Publications, Inc.

Senior Editor: Kristin Eclov
Editor: Christine Hood
Interior Design: Good Neighbor Press, Inc., Grand Junction, CO
Cover Illustration: Nancee McClure
Illustration: Janet Skiles and Kathryn Marlin

Fearon Teacher Aids products were formerly manufactured and distributed by American Teaching
Aids, Inc., a subsidiary of Silver Burdett Ginn, and are now manufactured and distributed by Frank
Schaffer Publications, Inc. FEARON, FEARON TEACHER AIDS, and the FEARON balloon logo are
marks used under license from Simon & Schuster, Inc.

© **Fearon Teacher Aids**
A Division of Frank Schaffer Publications, Inc.
23740 Hawthorne Boulevard
Torrance, CA 90505-5927

FE7959
ISBN 1-56417-974-5

TABLE OF CONTENTS

Table of Contents

Preparing Children for Everyday Dangers

What You Can Do to Help

The world is filled with dangers for children (and adults). Some are small dangers, like scraped knees, minor cuts and bruises. Some are major dangers, like having a child abducted or involved in a serious accident. As adults responsible for children, we want to protect them from all dangers, both minor and major. But we can't watch them every minute of every day. So we must do our best to prepare children at an early age to be aware of potentially dangerous situations, places, and people, and to protect themselves from harm.

The world is a scary place. Bad things happen. The dark side of reality is that natural disasters, strangers, and other potential threats to their safety and health are part of everyday life. Children must be aware of the dangers they face in the everyday world. We need to inform and prepare them without making them so afraid they become paranoid. No one wants to scare children. Many have enough fears already, real as well as imaginary. They have seen bad things happen on television. They may have watched scary movies. Worry about alien monsters might be stronger at this age than the fear of falling out of a tree or being hit by a car.

Children need to learn there are many dangers around them. Situations, objects, animals, people, and even plants can be dangerous. Fear can be healthy. Fear of a dark alley may keep a child from entering. Fear of falling out of a tree may keep a child from climbing too high. Fear encourages us to be careful. If children understand the potential dangers and are taught how to cope with them, they will be better prepared when confronted with these situations.

The bright side is that children can learn to handle most situations. You can teach them how. A child who is prepared has a better chance of growing up safe and happy. By preparing children in advance, we can help relieve many of the unnecessary fears they have.

First, we need to teach children awareness of potential dangers. Second, they need to learn how to handle those situations. It is not enough to give children a set of rules and expect them to follow them without question. They need to understand the basis for the rules and the reasons why safety rules are necessary.

Catch Them Doing Something Right!

Too often we remind children of what they do wrong and forget to praise them when they do something right. Everyone reacts more positively and gets more encouragement from praise than criticism.

To encourage the children in your class to practice good safety habits, make copies of the certificate on the next page on brightly-colored construction paper. Then, when you catch a child following a safety rule, present the certificate and praise him or her in front of the others. Fill in the lines with the specific safety rule that he or she followed. Encourage children to take their certificates home to share with their families.

v

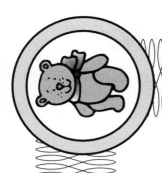
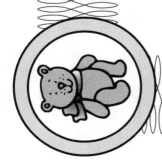

SAFETY AWARD

This safety award is presented to

for practicing good safety habits at school.

KEEP UP THE GOOD WORK!

(Teacher's signature)

(Date)

Using Safety for Young Children in Your Classroom

This book is divided into six major areas of safety. The first section covers general information for children, introduces the topic of safety, explains the meaning of an emergency, and gives children information about very basic first aid. The second section covers safety from strangers, at home, on the telephone, and in public places. Section three includes fire safety, family fire drills, and what to do in the event of a fire. The fourth section covers various areas of household safety. Outdoor safety and sports safety are addressed in the last two sections.

For most topics, one or more safety rules are introduced at the beginning of the section on that topic. For every safety rule, there is a reason, sometimes several reasons, included. When you discuss safety rules, ask children why they think it is a good rule. If they can think through and come up with reasons of their own, they will be more likely to remember the rule.

Following the rules section, you will find a short introduction to the topic related to the safety rules presented. This information can be relayed to children in your own words.

A discussion section follows. This allows children more opportunity to talk about the safety rules on a specific topic.

You will also find extension activities and reproducibles related to the topic in many sections. Take-home reproducibles reinforce the important home-school connection. Safety awareness must be a joint venture between parents and teachers.

Use children's books on related topics to supplement the safety topics you discuss in class. The following bibliography of easy-reading, colorfully illustrated safety books includes many sources you and the children will find useful and interesting.

General Safety Books for Children:

Dinosaurs, Beware: A Safety Guide by Marc Brown and Stephen Krensky. (Little, Brown and Company, 1982).

Every Kid's Guide to Responding to Danger by Joy Berry (Children's Press, 1987).

Henry Possum by Harold Berson (Crown, 1973).

Let's Find Out About Safety by Martha and Charles Shapp (Franklin Watts, 1975).

What to Do When Your Mom or Dad Says . . . Be Careful by Joy Wilt Berry (Children's Press, 1983).

Yes, No, Little Hippo by Jane Belk Mancure (Children's Press, 1988).

First Aid and Emergency Response Books for Children:

Barron's First Aid for Kids by Gary R. Fleicher, M.D. (Barron's International Series, Inc., 1987).

Help! Emergencies That Could Happen to You and How to Handle Them by Mary Lou Vandenburg (Lerner, 1975).

A Kid's Guide to First Aid: What Would You Do If . . . by Lory Freeman (Parenting Press, Inc., 1983).

Kids to the Rescue: First-Aid Techniques for Kids by Maribeth and Darwin Boelts (Parenting Press, Inc., 1992).

What to Do When There's No One But You by Harriet Margolis Gore (Prentice Hall, 1974).

Safety from Strangers Books for Children:

The Dangers of Strangers by Carole G. Vogel and Kathryn A. Goldner (Dillon Press, Inc., 1983).

Who Is a Stranger and What Should I Do? by Linda Walvoord Girard (Albert Whitman & Company, 1985).

Sports Safety Books for Children:

The Bear's Bicycle by Emilie McLeod (Little, 1975).

Driving Your Bike Safely by Corinne J. Naden (Julian Messner, 1979).

Lucky Chuck by Beverly Cleary (Morrow, 1984).

Who Tossed That Bat? Safety on the Ball Field and Playground by Leonard Kessler (Lothrop, Lee & Shepard Co., 1973).

Weather Safety Books for Children:

Flash, Crash, Rumble, and Roll by Franklyn M. Branley (Thomas Y. Crowell, 1985).

Hurricane Watch by Franklyn M. Branley (Thomas Y. Cromwell, 1985).

Tornado Alert by Franklyn M. Branley (Thomas Y. Crowell, 1988).

Fire and Household Safety Books for Children:

Dealing with Weapons at School and at Home by Lorelei Apel (Power Kids Press, 1996).

Fire by Cynthia Fitterer Klingel (Creative Eduction, 1986).

Safety Town books: Children's Press has produced a set of safety books for young children called the *Safety Town Series.* More information about Safety Town is included on the next page. Each book presents a safety concept through brightly-colored drawings and first person, easy-to-read text. Titles in this series include:

Animals Can Be Special Friends
Bicycles Are Fun to Ride
In the Water . . . On the Water
Matches, Lighters, and Firecrackers Are Not Toys
Playing on the Playground
Poisons Make You Sick
Riding On a Bus
Stop, Look, and Listen for Trains
Strangers
When I Cross the Street
When I Ride in a Car
When There is a Fire . . . Go Outside

Another excellent series of safety books for young children are published by Child's World. Titles in this series include:

Bicycle Safety	*Outdoor Safety*
Emergencies	*School Safety*
Fire Safety	*Traffic Safety*
Home Safety	*Water Safety*

Creative Education publishes a series called Safety First. Titles in this series include:

Bicycles	*Outdoors*
Fire	*School*
Home	*Water*

SAFETY TOWN

Safety Town is a comprehensive educational program that introduces safety awareness and preventive procedures to preschool children. During the 20-hour course, children learn, through their own involvement, safety rules about fire, poison, strangers, traffic, home, train, car, bus, playground, animals, toys, and other areas. They participate in safety activities in the classroom and practice safety lessons on an outdoor layout, which consists of a miniature town complete with houses, sidewalks, and crosswalks. Role-playing in simulated and real-life situations, under the guidance of a teacher and uniformed personnel, provides children with valuable learning experiences. This allows them to respond properly when confronted with potentially dangerous situations that occur in everyday life.

National Safety Town Center, established in 1964, is the pioneer organization dedicated to promoting preschool-early childhood safety education. This nonprofit organization has been largely responsible for enlightening the media, corporations, government officials, and the general public to the importance of safety education for children. Its network of dedicated volunteers continually supports and promotes the importance of safety for children through the Safety Town Program.

During the 20-hour, hands-on course (two hours per day for two weeks) children learn through their own involvement under the guidance of a teacher, uniformed personnel, and volunteer instructors. The course includes an indoor classroom where children observe and participate in safety activities through games, puzzles, stories, demonstrations, and artwork. The outdoor layout consists of a miniature town with houses, sidewalks, crosswalks, railroad crossings, and street markings. Here children practice and experience simulated situations so that they may respond decisively when confronted with similar situations in real life. Parent involvement is encouraged to provide supplemental learning at home. In 1997, 980 Safety Programs were in operation.

Safety Town has activity books, coloring books, card games, song tapes, and puzzles available to introduce and reinforce positive safety concepts for young children.

For additional information about the Safety Town Program, materials available, and how to establish a Safety Town in your community, contact the National Safety Town Center at P.O. Box 39312, Cleveland, Ohio 44139. Telephone (216) 831-7433.

WHY IS SAFETY IMPORTANT?

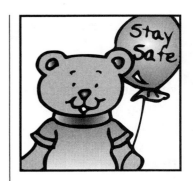

Introduction

Children face many dangers to their safety in everyday life. They may cross busy streets on their way to school. They ride in cars, buses, and on bikes. They take part in sports activities, go swimming, skating, and kite-flying. Children need to understand potential dangers and learn how to cope with them.

Discussion

How many times have you heard your parents or teachers say, "Be careful?" What does "Be careful" mean? Does it always mean the same thing?

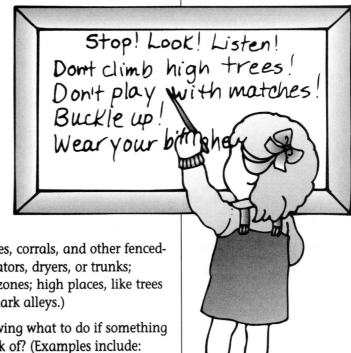

What does safety mean to you? Why is safety important to you, your friends, and family?

Safety means being careful with dangerous objects so no one gets hurt. What are some dangerous objects around your home? (Examples include: knives, electrical outlets, guns, power tools, cleaning products, lawn mowers, stairs, swings, stoves, microwaves, and swimming pools.)

Safety means avoiding dangerous places. What are some dangerous places where you need to be careful? Why are they dangerous, and what should you do about them? (Examples include: parking lots; animal enclosures, like cages, corrals, and other fenced-in areas; streets and highways; enclosed spaces, like refrigerators, dryers, or trunks; places where large machines are working, like construction zones; high places, like trees or ladders; big holes in the ground; deep water; caves, and dark alleys.)

Safety means being aware of dangerous situations and knowing what to do if something happens. What are some dangerous situations you can think of? (Examples include: natural disasters, like storms, tornadoes, hurricanes and floods; fires; car accidents; explosions; criminals, like robbers and kidnappers; encounters with wild or unfriendly animals.)

Activities

Write the words *Be Prepared* on the board. Ask children if this is a good safety slogan. Why or why not? ("Be prepared" is good advice, but a safety slogan should really be more specific.)

Ask children to brainstorm ideas for safety slogans that address specific situations, like *Always Wear Your Seatbelt* or *Don't Play with Matches*. Help them write their slogan ideas on banners to display in your classroom.

What Is an Emergency?

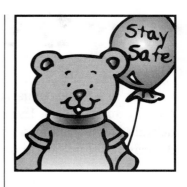

Introduction

Sometimes, no matter how careful we are, accidents happen. Accidents can be scary. Knowing what to do can make the situation less frightening. It's important to know what to do in an emergency to help yourself or someone else.

Discussion

Help children understand the difference between a minor accident, like a scraped knee, and a serious emergency by completing the following activity.

Is It an Emergency?

Ask children to answer "yes" or "no" to each question and explain their answers.

Is a fire an emergency?

If someone is badly burned, is that an emergency?

If someone breaks a bone, is that an emergency?

If someone gets bit by a mosquito, is that an emergency?

If someone is bleeding a lot, and you can't stop the bleeding, is that an emergency?

If someone can't breathe, is that an emergency?

If someone scrapes an elbow or a knee, is that an emergency?

If someone gets a piece of broken glass in his or her hand, is that an emergency?

What other examples of emergencies can you think of?

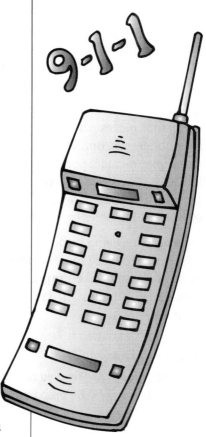

Activities

Teach children how to dial for help. In most places, 911 is the number to call in an emergency. If your community has another number, teach them that number.

When you call the emergency number you will need to give some information:

- type of emergency
- your name
- your address or where you are calling from

After you give that information, don't hang up. The person may want to tell you what to do until help arrives. Follow all instructions carefully.

Role-play emergency situations. Ask children to show what they would do. Have them use a toy telephone to dial the emergency number. You or another child can be the emergency person who answers.

See page 19 for a take-home list of emergency telephone numbers.

CHILDREN CAN LEARN FIRST AID

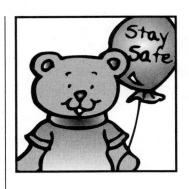

Introduction

Learning about first aid may seem like a big responsibility, and it is. Aid means help. Giving first aid means being the first person to help someone who is hurt. Knowing what to do for minor injuries can make someone feel better quickly. Knowing when to call for help may save a person's life or keep a bad injury from getting worse.

1. Know where first-aid supplies are kept in your house.

2. Know how to call for emergency help.

3. Keep calm. Take a deep breath. Don't panic.

Nobody expects you to know everything doctors and nurses do. Just do your best.

Words to Teach

injury, unconscious, hazardous, allergic

Discussion

Have you ever given first-aid to anyone? What happened? What did you do? Have you ever received first aid? What happened?

Activities

Invite someone from the American Red Cross or other medical personnel to give a "hands-on" demonstration of simple first-aid skills. Encourage children to participate.

Read each of the "what if" questions on pages 4–8 to the class. Talk about what to do in each situation. Do only one or two a day so children are not overwhelmed with too much information too quickly. Review what they've learned before going on to new topics.

Make copies of pages 4–8 for each child. Demonstrate each first-aid step shown, either with a child or a doll. Do no more than one page a day so children are not overwhelmed with too much information too quickly.

Ask children to make up other similar situations and talk about what they should do. Let them practice on each other, on dolls, or other action figures.

Make copies of pages 10–12 for children to take home and share with their parents. If possible, put pages 19 and 20 back to back in clear, plastic sheet protectors.

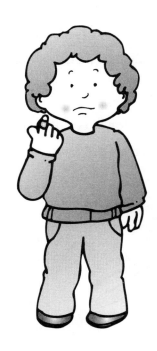

FIRST AID

Small Cuts

What would you do if you fell and cut your knee on a sharp stone?

1. Hold a clean towel or cloth tightly over the cut until the bleeding stops.

2. Clean the cut with soap and water.

3. Put on a bandage.

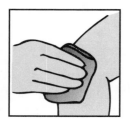 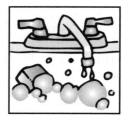 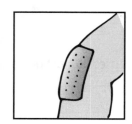

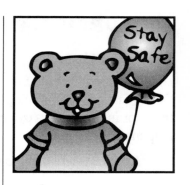

Deep or Large Cuts

What would you do if your dad fell on some broken glass and got a big, deep cut?

1. If someone is bleeding a lot, put a clean cloth on the area and press hard. Pressure helps stop bleeding.

2. Call for help.

3. Keep pressure on until help arrives.

4. Wash with soap and water.

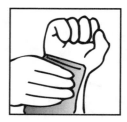 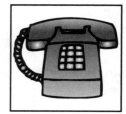 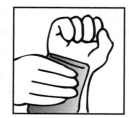 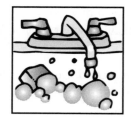

Slivers

What would you do if you were raking and got a sliver in your hand?

1. Pull out the sliver with clean tweezers.

2. Wash with soap and water.

3. Put on a bandage.

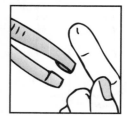 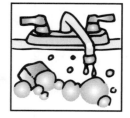 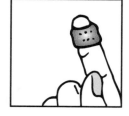

4

Bumps, Bruises, and Black Eyes

What would you do if you fell off a teeter-totter and bumped your head?

Put ice or a cool, wet washcloth on a bump, bruise, or black eye.

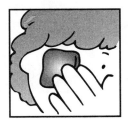

Nosebleeds

What would you do if your brother got bopped in the nose with a tennis ball and it started bleeding?

1. Have your brother sit down and lean forward.

2. Hold a dry washcloth firmly on the soft part of the nose for ten minutes.

3. Do not let your brother blow his nose.

4. If bleeding does not stop after ten minutes, call an adult to decide if your brother needs to go to the doctor.

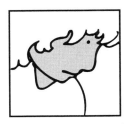 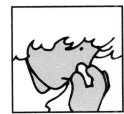 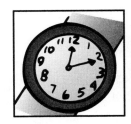 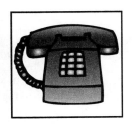

Broken Bones

What would you do if your sister fell off her bike and thought she had a broken arm?

If you think someone has a broken bone, keep that part of the body as still as possible while you call for help. Moving could make it worse.

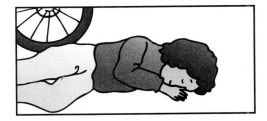

Insect Stings

What would you do if you were weeding the garden and got stung by a bee?

1. Put ice on an insect sting to keep the swelling down and stop it from itching.

2. Mix a few drops of water with a large spoonful of baking soda together to make a paste.

3. Cover the sting with the baking soda and water paste.

4. Have an adult check to see if the stinger is out. Remove the stinger with clean tweezers.

Usually insect stings are minor. Some people are very allergic to insect stings. If you or someone else is stung and has trouble breathing or faints, call for emergency help.

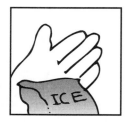  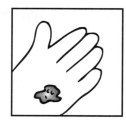 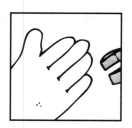

Eyes

What would you do if some bleach or other hazardous product splashed in your mother's eye?

1. Turn on the water in the sink so it is slightly warm.

2. Have your mother put her head under the faucet so the eye is under the running water. Have her hold the eye open. Do not rub it.

3. She should keep her eye under the running water for at least ten minutes.

4. Ask her to have a doctor check the eye.

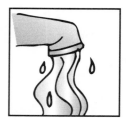 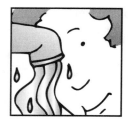  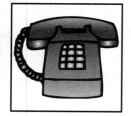

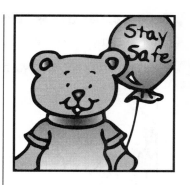

6

Eating or Drinking Poison

What would you do if your sister drank some cleaning liquid or other hazardous product?

1. If someone eats or drinks something that might be poisonous, call 911 or the emergency number in your area immediately.

2. Get the bottle of whatever your sister drank. The person who answers the emergency number needs to know what kind of poison, and if possible, how much she drank.

3. Follow the instructions given to you by the person who answers the phone.

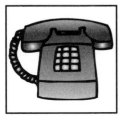 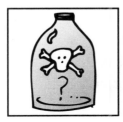 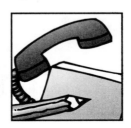

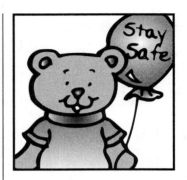

Poison Plants

What would you do if you were walking in the woods and suddenly started feeling itchy all over?

Some plants are poisonous and will cause a rash and itching.

1. Wash the area completely with soap and water.

2. You may have gotten some of the poison on your clothes also. Remove them and get them washed, too.

3. Try not to scratch. If the itching is very bad, put calamine lotion on the area.

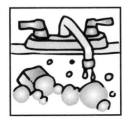 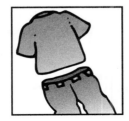 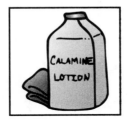

Lost Tooth

What would you do if you lost a tooth and your mouth was bleeding?

Hold a tissue on the spot for a few minutes until the bleeding stops.

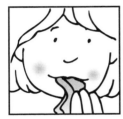

Minor Burns

What would you do if you burned your hand on a toaster?

Apply ice or a cool, wet washcloth to a small burn.

If a burn is serious or very large, call an adult or dial the number for emergency help.

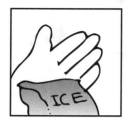

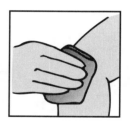

Animal Bites

What would you do if you were playing ball with the neighbor's dog, and it bit you by mistake when you reached for the ball?

1. A small bite by a dog or cat that breaks the skin should be treated like a minor cut.

2. Wash the area with soap and water.

3. Put on a bandage.

Always inform an adult if you have been bitten by an animal. If the animal has not had its shots, it will need to be watched for several days to make sure it is not sick.

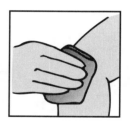 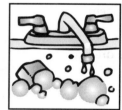 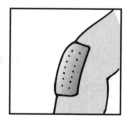

Serious Injuries

1. Call an adult in case of serious injury. Dial 911 or the emergency number in your area.

2. Don't move an unconscious person or anyone who is seriously hurt unless he or she is in danger.

3. Do what you can to stop any bleeding.

4. Sometimes after an injury, a person will suddenly feel very cold. Put a jacket or blanket around him or her until help arrives.

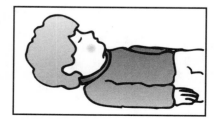 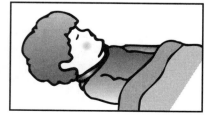

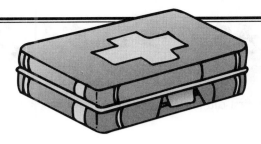

Dear Parents:

Do you have a first-aid kit in your home? Do you keep one in each car? If you have a boat or a cabin, do you keep one there, too? If you don't, now would be a good time to get one or more for your family's safety.

If you and your family go camping, hiking, fishing, or participate in other outdoor activities, do you have a first-aid kit to take along? If not, now is a good time to get one ready.

Does everyone in your family know where the first-aid kits are kept? If not, now is a good time to show them.

Have you checked in your first-aid kit lately to be sure it is fully stocked? If not, now is a good time to go through the supply checklist and refill the kit. You never know when you might need it.

Recommended First-Aid Supplies

_____ Scissors

_____ Sunscreen

_____ Thermometer

_____ Tweezers

_____ Needle to remove slivers

_____ Cleansing agent/soap

_____ Tongue depressors (2) These can also be used as small splints

_____ Moist towelettes

_____ Safety pins

_____ Triangular bandages (3)

_____ 2" sterile gauze pads (4 to 6)

_____ 4" sterile gauze pads (4 to 6)

_____ 3" sterile roller bandages (3 rolls)

_____ 4" sterile roller bandages (3 rolls)

_____ Sterile adhesive bandages in various sizes

_____ 2% hydrogen peroxide solution for use as disinfectant

_____ Laxatives

_____ Anti-diarrhea medication

_____ Aspirin or non-aspirin pain reliever

_____ Antacid

_____ Activated charcoal to use if advised by the Poison Control Center

_____ Syrup of ipecac to induce vomiting if advised by the Poison Control Center

_____ A first-aid manual or chart for reference

You can further protect your family by taking first aid and CPR courses sponsored by the American Red Cross.

Basic First Aid

Dear Parents:

Please keep this chart and your first-aid kit in a place where everyone can find them quickly.

Small Cuts

1. Hold a clean towel or cloth tightly over the cut until the bleeding stops.

2. Clean the cut with soap and water.

3. Put on a bandage.

Deep or Large Cuts

1. If someone is bleeding a lot, put a clean cloth on the area and press hard. Pressure helps stop bleeding.

2. Call for help.

3. Keep pressure on until help arrives.

Slivers

1. Pull out slivers with clean tweezers.

2. Wash with soap and water.

3. Put on a bandage.

Bumps, Bruises, and Black Eyes

Apply ice or a cool, wet washcloth to the area to reduce swelling. (Cuts near the eye may need to be checked by a doctor.)

Nosebleeds

1. Have the person sit down and lean forward.

2. Hold a dry washcloth firmly on the soft part of the nose for ten minutes.

3. Do not let the person blow his or her nose.

4. If bleeding does not stop after ten minutes, call a doctor.

Broken Bones

If you think someone has a broken bone, keep that part of the body as still as possible while you call for help. Moving could make it worse.

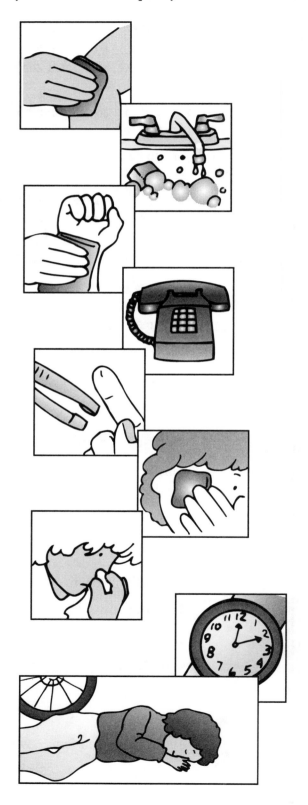

Reproducible

BASIC FIRST AID

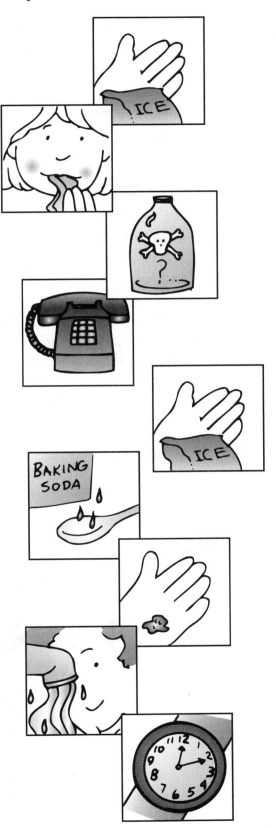

Minor Burns

Apply ice or a cool, wet washcloth to a small burn.

If a burn is serious or very large, dial the number for emergency help.

Lost Tooth

Hold a tissue on the spot for a few minutes until the bleeding stops.

Eating or Drinking Poison

1. If someone eats or drinks something that might be poisonous, call 911 or the emergency number in your area.

2. The person who answers will need to know what kind of poison, and if possible, how much the person ate or drank.

3. Follow the instructions given to you by the person who answers the phone.

Insect Stings

1. Put ice on an insect sting to keep the swelling down and stop it from itching.

2. Mix a few drops of water with a large spoonful of baking soda together to make a paste.

3. Cover the sting with the baking soda and water paste.

4. Check to see if the stinger is out. If not, remove the stinger with clean tweezers.

Usually insect stings are minor. However, some people are very allergic to insect stings. If someone is stung and has trouble breathing or faints, call for emergency help.

Eyes

1. Turn on the water in the sink so it is slightly warm.

2. Have the person put his or her head under the faucet so the eye is under the running water. Have him or her hold the eye open. Do not rub it.

3. Keep warm running water on the eye for at least ten minutes.

4. Call a doctor to check the eye.

Basic First Aid

Poison Ivy, Oak, and Sumac

Some plants are poisonous and will cause rashes and itching.

1. Wash the area completely with soap and water.

2. Some of the poison may be on the clothes also. Remove them and get them washed, too.

3. If the itching is very bad, put calamine lotion on the area.

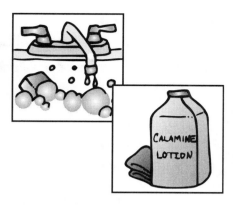

Animal Bites

1. A small bite by an animal that breaks the skin should be treated like a minor cut.

2. If the animal has not had its shots, it will need to be watched for several days to make sure it is not sick.

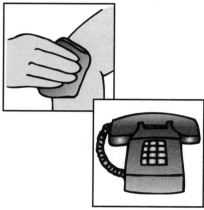

Serious Injuries

1. Call for emergency help when a serious injury occurs. Dial 911 or the emergency number in your area.

2. Don't move an unconscious person or anyone who is seriously hurt he or she is in danger.

3. Do what you can to stop any bleeding.

4. Sometimes after an injury, a person will suddenly feel very cold. Put a jacket or blanket around him or her until help arrives.

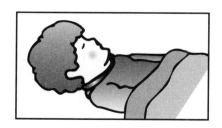

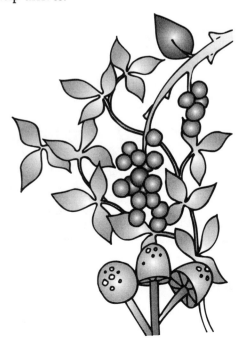

Reproducible

SAFETY FROM STRANGERS

ACCEPTING RIDES AND GIFTS FROM STRANGERS

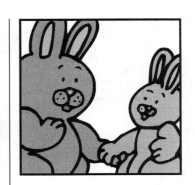

The Rules	The Reason
Never ride or walk anywhere with ANYONE unless your parents have told you ahead of time that it's OK.	Some strangers are bad people and may want to hurt you.
Never leave a public building with a stranger.	Some people may try to hurt children or take them away from their parents.
Never accept gifts or money from strangers.	Some bad people try to trick children by offering them gifts or money.

What to Do

If a stranger asks you to go for a walk or get in a car, shout NO! and run away.

If a stranger offers you money or presents, shout NO! and run away.

Where should you run? Don't run off by yourself or try to hide in a place where there are no people. Run to a place where there are lots of people. Run into a restaurant or a gas station. Run to the home of someone you know well. Make a lot of noise. A bad stranger will not want anyone to see him or her. Making a lot of noise is good.

Introduction

Who is a stranger? A stranger is someone you do not know well. You have met many strangers already. Some have become friends. There are strangers in your neighborhood, in stores, and at school. Even people you see often, but don't really know, are strangers, like the mail carrier, the school bus driver, and the clerk at the store. Most strangers are nice people. They are helpful and friendly.

Some strangers are not good people. They may want to hurt a child or take him or her away from his or her parents. They may want to touch a child in ways that are not proper. Strangers don't become friends just by acting friendly for a few minutes.

Do you know the person's name? where he or she lives? Do your parents know that person? Do they trust that person?

Bad people do not always look mean or bad. They can seem to be friendly. They can be men or women, young or old. They can be dressed in grubby old clothes or in brand-new fancy ones.

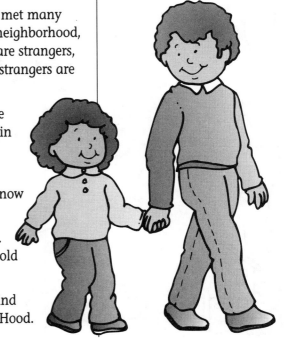

Remember the story of Little Red Riding Hood? The wolf pretended to be kind and friendly, but he was really mean. He wanted to hurt Little Red Riding Hood.

All About Me

My First Name is _____

My Last Name is _____

I Live at _____

_____

_____

My Apartment Number is _____

My City is _____

My State is _____

My Area Code is _____

My Telephone Number is _____

This is what I would say if a stranger wanted me to walk or ride somewhere.

No! No! No!

Safety from Strangers

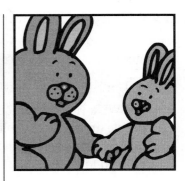

The Rules	The Reason
Do not talk to strangers when you are alone or with your friends.	Bad strangers may try to talk to you so you think they are friends. They may try to get close to you while you are talking.
Always go into public bathrooms with another child or an adult. Never go into a deserted bathroom at an empty place.	
If you see a stranger hanging around your school or playground, tell a teacher or another adult.	

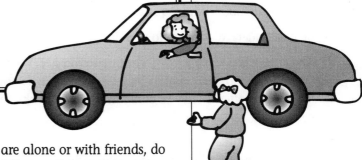

What to Do

If a stranger tries to stop you and asks questions when you are alone or with friends, do NOT answer. Leave the area immediately. If you are in a public building, go where there are other people. If you are outside, go to a place where there are people. Always tell your parents, teacher, a police officer, or someone you trust what happened as soon as possible.

Introduction

When you are with your parents and a stranger says, "Hi, how are you" it's OK to answer. When you are in the checkout line at a grocery store with your parents or an adult and the cashier says, "What a pretty blouse you have on," or "That's a neat cap," it's OK to answer politely because you are with your parents.

Role Play

A young man wearing jeans and a football jersey stops you and asks you questions, like: *What is your name? Where do you live?* He looks a lot like your favorite football player.

Is he a stranger? What should you do?

ANSWER: He is a stranger. Do not answer any questions about yourself. Get away from him fast. Go to a place where there are other people.

Role Play

You and your best friend are walking to the park. A woman asks you if the two of you would like to go with her to see a movie. She says she will buy popcorn and soda for you both.

Is she a stranger? What should you do?

ANSWER: She is a stranger. Shout, NO! Do not go ANYWHERE with her, even though you are with a friend. Leave the area immediately. Go to a place where there are other people. Tell an adult what happened. Never go anywhere with a stranger no matter what he or she says or offers you.

Role Play

A man who looks a lot like your grandfather tells you he is lost. He asks you to walk with him to the corner of Second and Maple Street, which is a few blocks away.

Is he a stranger? What should you do?

ANSWER: He is a stranger. Do not go ANYWHERE with him. If there are other people around, you could ask someone else to help the man. If no one else is around, stay away from the man. Tell him you are sorry, but you aren't allowed to do that. Most adults ask other adults for help, not children.

Role Play

A lady stops you and says, "Will you come with me and help me find my dog? I will give you $10. I know my poor little dog is so scared." She starts to cry.

Is she a stranger? What should you do?

ANSWER: She is a stranger. You should not go ANYWHERE with her. If other people are around, ask them to help her. This lady is not acting right. Most adults will not offer money to children. They will ask other adults to help.

Role Play

A man calls out from an alley and asks for your help. He looks like he is bleeding.

Is he a stranger? What should you do?

ANSWER: He is a stranger. Do not go close to him. He may be pretending. Call loudly for help. Get another adult to help. Use the nearest telephone and call the emergency number.

Role Play

A young man about 20 years old driving a fancy red convertible stops his car in front of your house and asks you for directions.

Is he a stranger? What should you do?

ANSWER: He is a stranger. Don't go near the car. Usually adults ask other adults for directions, not children.

Role Play

You are shopping with your mother at a large department store. You wander off to the toy aisle. A man in a store uniform comes up to you and says, "Hurry, your mom fell and broke her leg. The ambulance took her to the hospital. I'll take you there."

Is he a stranger? What should you do?

ANSWER: He is a stranger. Do not go with him. How would he know she was your mother? If she really did have a broken leg, someone would make an announcement for you to come to the front desk. Go to the front desk and find out if anything really did happen to your mother.

It's best if you stay with your parents when shopping. If you do wander off alone, do not leave the store or go somewhere else in the store with a stranger.

16

Telephone Strangers

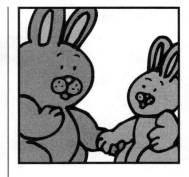

The Rules	The Reason
Never tell a caller that you are home alone or with a sitter. If you do not know the person who is calling, do not answer ANY questions.	A bad stranger might try to come to your house if he or she knows your parents aren't home.

What to Do

If you don't know who is calling, ask the person to leave a message. You can say, "My mom can't come to the phone right now. Can you leave a message?"

Role Play *with a toy telephone*

When you answer the phone, a lady says she is calling from your school and needs some information. She wants you to answer questions.

> Is she a stranger? What should you do?

> ANSWER: She is a stranger. If you are alone, ask her to call back later or offer to take a message. If your parents are home, ask her to wait while you get them. Do not answer any questions.

Role Play *with a toy telephone*

You are home alone and the phone rings. When you answer, it is your grandmother. She wants to talk to your dad.

> Is she a stranger? What should you do?

> ANSWER: She is not a stranger. It's OK to tell her your dad isn't home. It's OK to answer questions about when he will be back. Offer to take a message. Don't forget to give your dad the message.

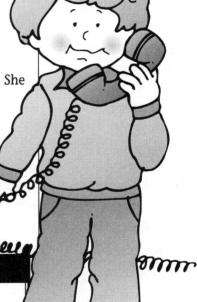

Strangers at Your Door

The Rules	The Reason
Always ask who is there before you open the door. If you do not know the person, do NOT open the door.	A stranger might try to get into your home to hurt you or to steal things.

What to Do

If your parents aren't home, NEVER let strangers into the house. Don't tell them you are alone. Ask them to come back later.

If you don't know who is at the door, and your parents are home, ask the person to please wait while you go get them. Don't let strangers into your home even if your parents are there.

If a stranger won't go away and keeps ringing or knocking, call a neighbor or call the police. It's never wrong to ask for help.

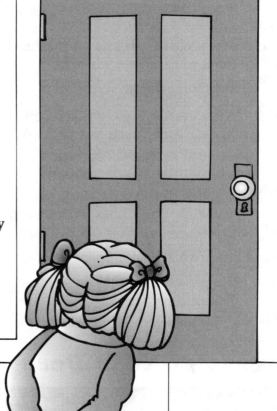

Role Play

Someone knocks on the door and says, "I'm a police officer, let me in."

Is this a stranger? What should you do?

ANSWER: This is a stranger. Don't open the door. Call your parents to come to the door if they are home. Don't tell the person you are alone. Ask them to come back later. Sometimes bad strangers dress up in uniforms and pretend to be police officers, people who work for the power company, or delivering packages.

Role Play

Someone rings your doorbell. "Flowers for Mrs. Brown," says a voice.

Is this a stranger? What should you do?

ANSWER: This is a stranger. Don't open the door. Call your parents to come to the door if they are home. If they are not home, ask the person to leave the flowers by the door or come back later. Do NOT tell the person you are alone.

Role Play

Someone knocks on your door. "Help me!" he shouts. "I had an accident and I'm hurt."

Is this a stranger? What should you do?

ANSWER: This is a stranger. Don't open the door if you are alone. Dial the emergency number. Tell the person who answers what is going on. If your parents are home, call them to come to the door immediately. Sometimes bad people pretend to need help so you will let them in your house.

EMERGENCY NUMBERS

FIRE:_____

POLICE:_____

AMBULANCE:_____

DOCTOR:_____

DENTIST:_____

POISON CONTROL CENTER:_____

RESPONSIBLE ADULTS TO CALL

NAME

NUMBER

_____ _____

_____ _____

_____ _____

_____ _____

To Parents: Please fill in the above information. Make copies of this sheet and hang one copy near each telephone in your house. This will help your children or sitters respond quickly to an emergency. Review with your children when and how to call for help.

It is important that children know their telephone number, including area code, and their complete address, including city and state. Write this information below and review it with your children.

OUR TELEPHONE NUMBER

(_____) _____

OUR ADDRESS

STREET # _____

CITY _____

STATE/ZIP _____

WHAT WOULD YOU DO?

The next six pages illustrate various scenarios with children and strangers. Make copies for each child. Read the text below each picture to the class. Let children study the picture and take turns suggesting what to do in each situation. Encourage them to suggest other similar situations and what the proper response would be.

Responses to the situations should include the following:

A. This person is a stranger. Leave immediately and go tell a teacher.

B. She is a stranger. Shout, "No!" and run away. Run to the nearest place with lots of other people around. A woman who lost her little girl shouldn't be asking a child for help. She should be asking the police and other adults.

C. She is a stranger. Your parents are with you, there are other people around, and the person is giving pizza samples to everyone. It's OK to take one and say, "Thank you."

D. She is a stranger. You should shout, "No!" and run away.

E. He is a stranger. Say, "No," and go quickly to where your parents or other people are in the store.

F. She is a stranger. Say, "No," and look for a museum guard. Ask for help only from someone who works for the museum.

G. He is a stranger. Since you are with your parents, you can answer his question about the Packers.

H. This is a stranger. Do not open the door. You could ask the person to wait while you call your dad or ask the delivery person to come back in 15 minutes.

I. He is a stranger. You should not go with him unless he gives you the code word. You should tell your teacher. You could call your dad at work and check it out.

J. He is a stranger. You should go back inside by your parents immediately and tell them what happened.

K. In this case, it depends. If the neighbor is a good friend of your family's, it might be all right to accept a ride. If you don't know the person well, or aren't sure, say, "Thank you, no." It's better to be wet and safe. Talk to your parents about who you can accept rides from.

L. The person on the phone is a stranger. Do not give out any information, even if the person promises you a gift. Ask the person to wait while you get your mother or to call back later.

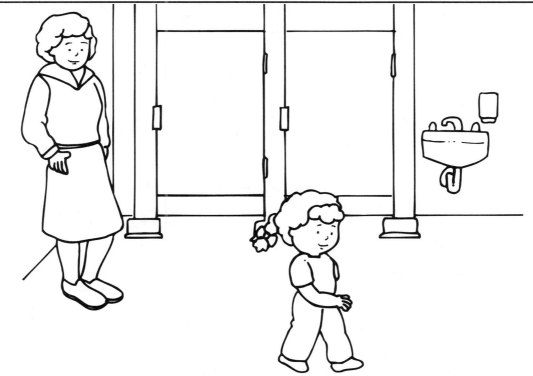

A. When you go in the bathroom at school, there is an adult there that isn't a teacher or anyone you know. The person isn't doing anything wrong, just hanging around.

Is this person a stranger? What should you do?

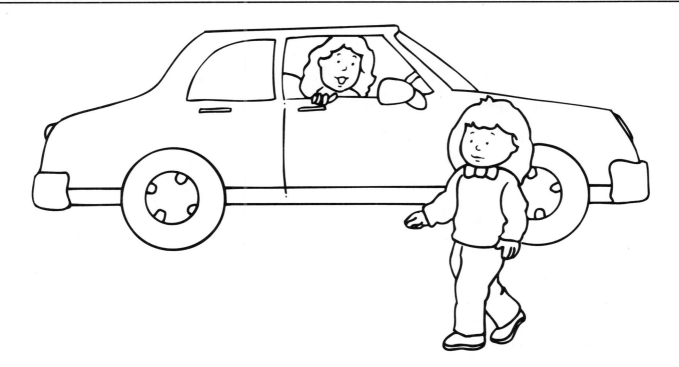

B. You are walking to the store. A pretty lady stops her car and asks for your help finding her missing little girl.

Is she a stranger? What should you do?

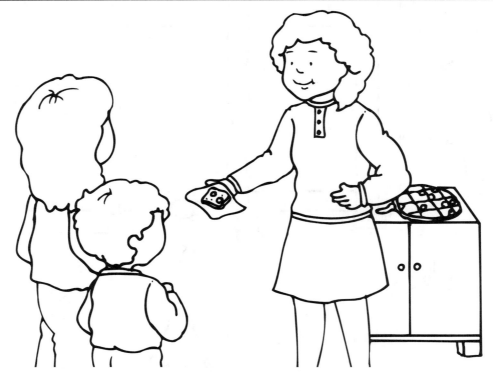

C. You're at the grocery store with your mom or dad. A lady is giving away free samples of pizza and offers you one.

Is she a stranger? What should you do?

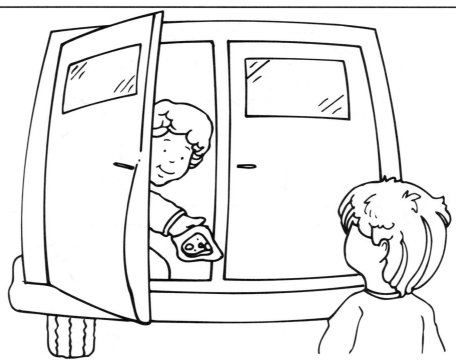

D. The next day you see the same lady driving down the street in a van. She recognizes you and pulls over. She opens the back door of the van and says, "I have more free samples of that pizza you liked. Come here, and I'll give you one."

Is she a stranger? What should you do?

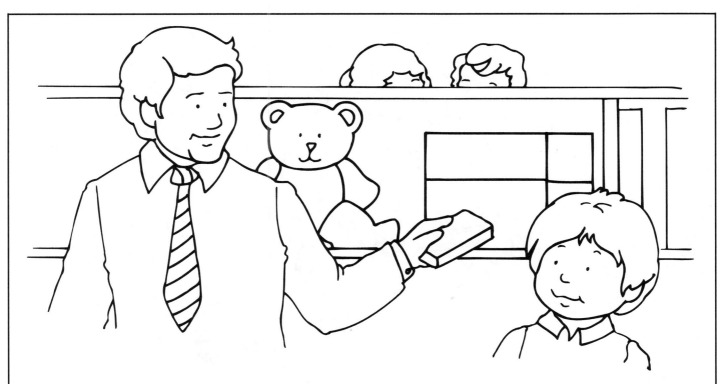

E. You're at the toy store. Your parents are in another aisle. A man says, "I'm giving away free samples of new, super video games to see how kids like them. Come out to my car and I'll give you one."

    Is he a stranger? What should you do?

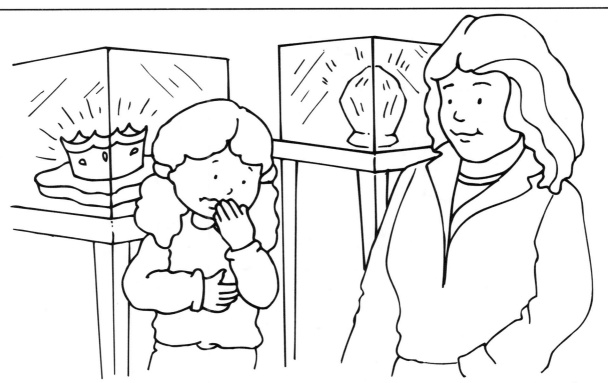

F. You're at the museum on a field trip with your class, and you get lost. A woman sees you are lost and offers to help you find your class.

    Is she a stranger? What should you do?

Reproducible

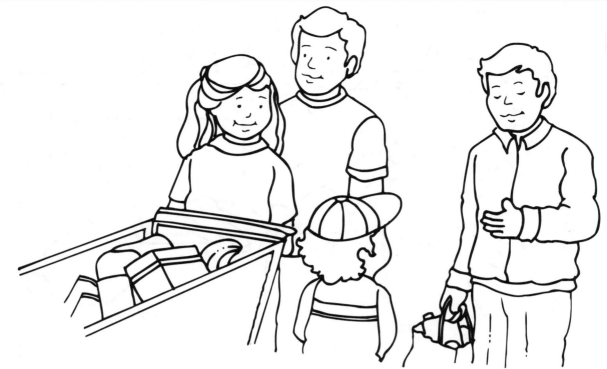

G. You're standing in line at the grocery checkout with your parents. The man behind you says, "I see you're wearing a Packers cap. They're my favorite team. Are they yours, too?"

Is this man a stranger? What should you do?

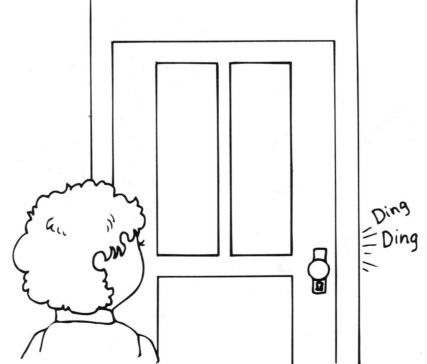

H. Your dad is upstairs taking a shower, and the doorbell rings. "Who's there?" you ask. "Special delivery for Mr. Brown," answers a voice. "Open the door so you can sign for the package."

Is this a stranger? What should you do?

Reproducible

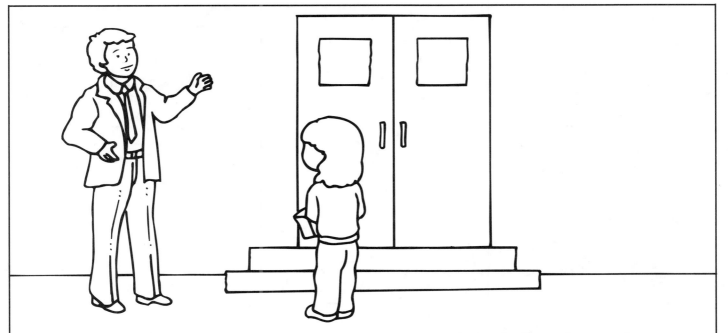

I. A man wearing a business suit and tie comes up to you after school and calls you by name, but you don't know him.

"I work with your dad," he says. "He told me to pick you up and take you to the baseball game. He'll meet us there."

Is he a stranger? What should you do?

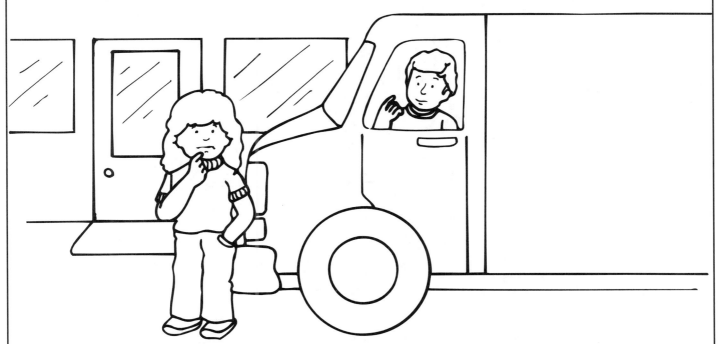

J. You walk outside to the parking lot from a restaurant while your parents are still inside paying the bill. A truck driver waves to you from across the parking lot. "How would you like to see inside my truck?" he asks.

Is he a stranger? What should you do.

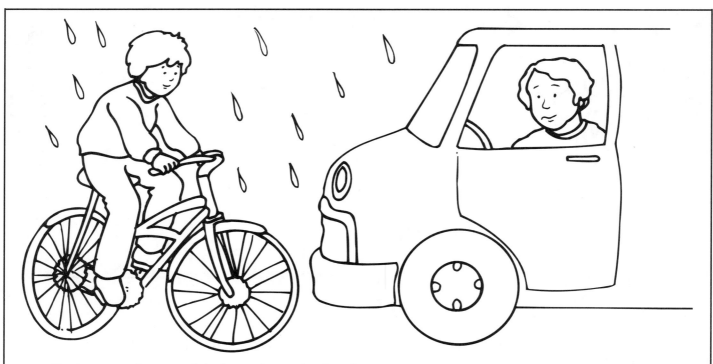

K. You are riding your bike home from school in the rain. A man you've seen in the neighborhood stops his car. He offers to put your bike in the truck and give you a ride home. You are cold and wet and miserable.

Is he a stranger? What should you do?

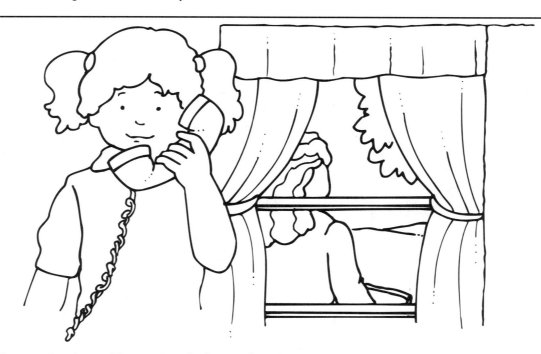

L. Your mother is outside mowing the lawn. The telephone rings and you answer politely. "Hi," says a voice you don't know. "I'm taking a survey to find out how many children watch the 'Clarence, the Clown Show'. We will send prizes to all children who answer our questions. If you watch 'Clarence, the Clown', tell me your name and address and how old you are."

Is this a stranger? What should you do?

Sexual and Physical Abuse of Children

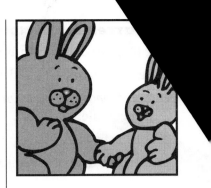

Many communities have organizations set up to teach children how to say NO to uncomfortable situations. They use puppets, stories, videos, and illustrations to emphasize to children that they do not have to keep secrets about sexual or physical abuse, and that help is available.

Teaching children how to protect themselves from strangers is one way to prevent sexual abuse. However, a study by the Planned Parenthood League showed that at least 75% of sexual abuse cases involved an adult the child knew and trusted like a doctor, teacher, coach, sitter, neighbor, or relative.

If a child reports an incident of sexual or physical abuse to you, take the child seriously. Children rarely lie about this.

Some schools have specific programs for dealing with this problem and specific people designated to teach this sensitive subject. Check with your local police station, hospital, Social Services Department, or other local organizations to find resources in your community. Although these two specific topics are not included in this book, a list of resources for children and adults is included below.

Resources for Children

All Alone After School by Muriel Stanek (Albert Whitman, 1984).

A Better Safe Than Sorry Book by Sol and Judith Gordon (Ed-U Press, Inc., 1984).

My Body Is Private by Linda Walvoord Girard (Albert Whittman, 1984).

Help Yourself to Safety: A Guide to Avoiding Dangerous Situations with Strangers and Friends by Kate Hubbard and Evelyn Berlin (The Charles Franklin Press, 1985).

It's My Body: A Book to Teach Young Children How to Resist Uncomfortable Touch by Lory Freeman (Parenting Press, 1982).

It's Not Your Fault by Judy Jance (Kids Rights, 1985).

My Very Own Book About Me by Jo Stowell and Mary Dietzel (Spokane Rape Crisis Center, 1980).

My Very Own Special Body Book by Kerry Basset (Hawthorne Press, 1980).

No More Secrets for Me by Oralee Wachter (Little Brown and Co., 1994).

Once I Was a Little Bit Frightened by J. William (Rape and Abuse Crisis Center of Fargo-Moorhead, 1980).

Private Zone: Teaching Children Sexual Assault Prevention Tools by Frances S. Dayee (Warner Books, 1982).

Safety Zone: A Book Teaching Children Abduction Prevention Skills by Linda D. Meyer (The Charles Franklin Press, 1982).

What If I Say NO!! by Jill Haddad and Lloyd Martin (M.H Cap & Co.).

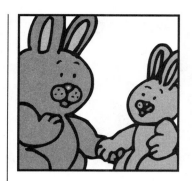

for Teachers and Parents

...buse Crisis Center, Fargo, ND, 1985).

...Sexual Abuse of Children by Florence Rush (Prentice-Hall, 1980).

...ence: Incest and Its Devastation by Susan Forward and Craig Buck ...guin Books, 1978).

Child Abuse by Stacey L. Tipp (Greenhaven Press, 1991).

Child Lures: A Guide to Prevent Abduction by Ken Wooden (Summit Publishing Group, June 1995).

The Common Secret: Sexual Abuse of Children and Adolescents by C. Henry Kemp, (W.H. Freeman and Co., 1995).

Conspiracy of Silence: The Trauma of Incest by Sandra Butler (New Glide Publications, 1978).

Cry Softly: The Story of Child Abuse by Margaret O. Hyde (Westminster Press, 1986).

Everything You Need to Know About Family Violence by Evan Stork (Roen Publishing Group, 1991).

He Told Me Not to Tell (King County Rape Relief, 1979).

Hidden Victims: The Sexual Abuse of Children by Robert L. Geiser (Beacon Press, 1979).

Kiss Daddy Goodnight: A Speakout on Incest by Louise Armstrong (Hawthorne Books, 1978).

My Body Is Mine, My Feelings Are Mine: A Storybook About Body Safety for Young Children with an Adult Guidebook by Susan Hoke (The Center for Applied Psychology, Inc., 1995).

Never Say Yes to a Stranger: What Your Child Must Know to Stay Safe by Susan Newman (Perigee Books, 1985).

New Strategies for Free Children: A Guide to Child Assault Prevention by Sally Cooper (National Assault Prevention Center, August, 1991).

No More Secrets: Protecting Your Child from Sexual Assault by Caren Adams and Jennifer Fay (Impact Publishers, 1981).

Protect Your Child from Sexual Abuse: A Parent's Guide 'A Book to Teach Young Children How to Resist Uncomfortable Touch'; by Janie Hart-Rossi (Planned Parenthood of Snohomish County, 1984).

Sexually Victimized Children by David Finkelhor (Free Press, 1979).

The Silent Children: A Book for Parents About the Prevention of Child Abuse by Linda Tschirhart Sanford (Anchor Press/Doubleday, 1980).

We Have a Secret by Lloyd Martin and Jill Haddad (Cap & Company, 1982).

Your Children Should Know by Flora Colao and Tamar Hosansky (Bobbs-Merrill, 1983).

Your Child's Self-Esteem by Dorothy Corkbille Briggs (Doubleday & Company, Inc., 1970)

Other Resources

Missing Children Network Hotline: 1-800-235-3535

National Child Abuse Hotline: 1-800-422-4453

National Coalition Against Domestic Violence: Box 15127, Washington, DC 20003-0127. Hotline: 1-800-333-SAFE

Survivors of Incest Anonymous: Box 21817, Baltimore, MD 21222

FIRE SAFETY
STOP! DROP! ROLL!

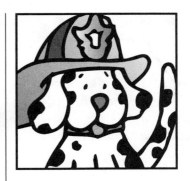

The Rule	The Reason
If your hair or clothing catches on fire, don't run.	Running will make the fire worse. Remember these three steps: **Stop! Drop! Roll!** Stop! Drop to the ground! Start rolling to put out the fire!

Introduction

Fires need air. Running gives fire more air, so it can grow bigger. By rolling on the ground, you can put out a fire. If a person's hair or clothing catches fire, you can help by shouting, "Stop! Drop! Roll!" Use a blanket or throw rug to help smother the fire.

Discussion

If your dad was cooking hamburgers on the grill and his barbecue apron caught on fire, what should he do? What are the three words to remember if someone's hair or clothing catches on fire?

Activity

On gym mats or outdoors on the grass, have children practice the Stop, Drop, and Roll. Show them how to use a blanket or throw rug to smother a fire.

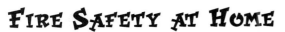

FIRE SAFETY AT HOME

The Rule	The Reason
If a door is door is closed and you smell smoke, don't open the door.	If you open the door, the fire and smoke will get in more quickly.

Introduction

If you smell smoke, it means there is a fire somewhere near. Feel the door. If it is hot, do not open it. A door gives you some protection from smoke and fire, at least for a little while. Look for another way to get out of the room.

Discussion

Why is it a good idea to sleep with your bedroom door closed? Are all fires bad? When is a fire good? (Campfires and grills are two examples of good fires.)

The Rule	The Reason
If a door is open, but fire or heavy smoke is blocking your way to the exit, shout for help out the window.	Firefighters will help you get out through a window safely.

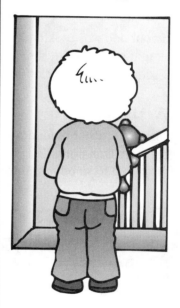

Introduction

The word EXIT means the way out of a room. Don't break the window and jump out unless you have no other choice. A fall from a high window could injure you.

The Rules	The Reason
Never try to hide from a fire.	Under the bed or in the closet is not a good place to go in a fire. You may be trapped there.
If you wake at night and smell smoke, call loudly to wake your family, then leave as quickly as possible.	By calling out, your family will be aware of the danger, too.
Go to a neighbor's and call for help.	Never stay in a building that is burning, not even long enough to call the fire deparment. You are in too much danger if you stay.
If you live in an apartment, never use an elevator during a fire.	If the power goes out, the elevator will stop working. Know where to find the stairs and fire exits.

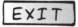

Introduction

Get outside as quickly as possible. Call to alert others in the house. Don't stop to take your favorite things. Don't stop to call the fire department. You may be trapped by the fire. Call for help from a neighbor's phone.

Discussion

Why shouldn't you take time to gather up your favorite toys? If you are wearing pajamas, should you take time to change into different clothes before you leave? Why should you go to a neighbor's house to call the fire department?

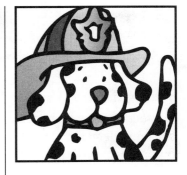

The Rule	The Reason
If heavy smoke is making you cough, crawl along the floor.	Smoke rises. The air is easier to breathe close to the floor.

Activity

Use chairs or empty cardboard boxes to form a path for children to crawl through. Mark one end with the word *FIRE* in large red letters. Mark the other end *EXIT*. Take yarn and crisscross it between the chairs about three feet off the ground. Tell children the yarn represents smoke. Remind children to keep low as they crawl so they don't get into the "smoke."

The Rule	The Reason
Have smoke detectors on every level in your home and in the garage, too. Test them monthly to be sure they are working.	Smoke detectors warn you by making a loud noise when there is smoke.

Discussion

Do you have smoke detectors in your home? How do smoke detectors warn you if there is a fire?

Activity

Bring a smoke detector to class. Show children how to test the smoke detector to see if it is working. (Let others in the school know when you will be testing the smoke detector, so they do not think it is a real fire.)

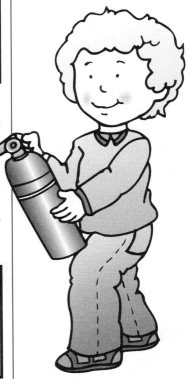

The Rule	The Reason
Never put water on a grease fire or an electrical fire. Use a fire extinguisher.	Water will make the fire spread faster.

Introduction

A grease fire could start if you were heating oil in a pan on the stove and it got too hot. An electrical fire could start if too many cords were plugged into one outlet, or from a cord that was broken. These types of fires cannot be put out with water.

What to Do

If a small fire starts in a pan on the stove, shut off the stove. Put a cover on the pan. Use the fire extinguisher if that doesn't put out the fire. If the fire is big, don't try to put it out yourself. Call for help. Leave and call the fire department from a neighbor's house.

Discussion

Do you have fire extinguishers in your house? Do you know how to use them? If there is a big fire, should you try to put it out yourself with a fire extinguisher?

Activity

Contact your local fire department. Invite them to present a fire safety program to your class and demonstrate the use of fire extinguishers. Encourage children to ask questions and participate in the discussion.

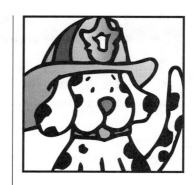

Family Fire Plan

Introduction

At home, you and your family should have a fire plan. A fire plan lets everyone know what to do and where to go if a fire starts in your house.

Practice your plan. Know two exits from every room, including the basement. Hold family fire drills.

Have a planned meeting place outside for your family. You'll know quickly if anyone is missing.

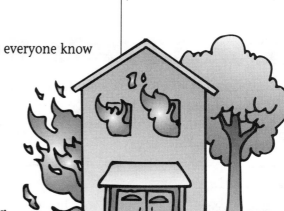

Discussion

Does your family have a fire plan? Will you tell us about your plan? Why is it a good idea to practice your family fire plan before a fire starts?

Do you ever spend the night at a friend's house or with relatives? Why should you ask them about their family fire plan? If they do not have one, what can you do?

Activity

Show children a floor plan of their classroom and the hallway to the fire exit. Ask children to draw a picture of the floor plan of their houses or apartments and mark their bedrooms. They can use arrows to show two ways to leave their bedrooms.

Fire Safety at School

The Rule	The Reason
If the fire alarm rings at school, leave the building at once. Walk, don't run.	It is important to leave a building quickly if a fire starts. If you run, you may trip and fall. Other children may fall, too.

Introduction

It is important to go a specific place outside so your teacher can check that everyone is safe. Tell children, "Our class should go to (NAME THE SPECIFIC LOCATION). If you are in the bathroom or someplace else outside the classroom when the fire alarm rings, go to this place so we will know you are safe."

32

Activities

Are there fire extinguishers at your school? Show children where they are and where to find the fire-alarm boxes. Explain what a child should do if he or she is the first one to spot a fire at school.

Hold a fire drill with your class. Explain to students what they should do and where they should go if the fire alarm rings when they are outside before or after school, or at recess.

Take a walk around the inside of the school. Have children point out all the EXIT signs they can find. Show them how to get to the closest exit from various places in the building, like the gym, bathrooms, and lunchroom.

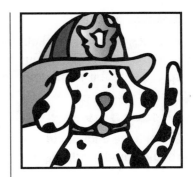

Fire Safety in Public Buildings

The Rules	The Reason
If fire starts in a public place, like a store or movie theater, leave immediately. Look for the red EXIT sign. Walk, don't run. Don't panic.	Walk quickly, but do not run. You may fall and trip if you run. You may cause other people to fall, too.
Never use an elevator during a fire.	During a fire, the power may go out and the elevators will stop working. You could be trapped.

Activity

The next time you take your class on a field trip, point out the EXIT signs in the building. Ask them to look for EXIT signs during trips with their parents to the mall, library, museum, etc.

Preventing Fires

The Rules	The Reason
Never play with matches, candles, or lighters.	Matches, lit candles, and lighters can start fires.
Keep rags and paper away from heat sources, like fireplaces, space heaters, and furnaces.	Rags and paper can catch fire easily and burn quickly. A small fire can quickly become a big one.
Never hang clothes on a space heater or wood-burning stove.	They may start a fire.
Empty the lint filter in the clothes dryer.	This keeps the airway clean and prevents fire.

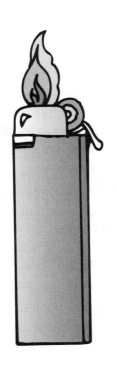

Introduction

Matches, candles, and lighters are not bad. They can be very useful at times. But they can also be very dangerous because they can start fires. Fires can burn you. Fires can spread. Fires burn buildings, people, and forests.

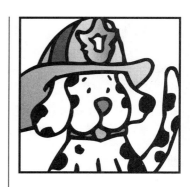

Discussion

If you have a lot of old newspapers or rags stored in your basement or garage, what should you do with them?

When do people need to use matches, lighters, and candles? Who should use matches and lighters? Where should matches and lighters be kept? Are matches toys? What should you do if you find matches or lighters? What should you do if you see another child playing with matches?

Read this poem to your class:

> *It is not good.*
> *It is not right.*
> *To read in bed*
> *By candlelight.*

Is this good fire-prevention advice? Why?

Activity

Ask children to make up their own short poems about fire safety or fire prevention.

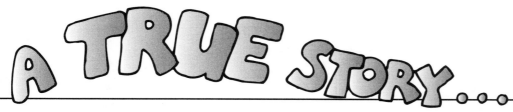

Jean lived in an apartment heated by oil space heaters. When she took clothes out of the dryer, sometimes they weren't quite dry. Then she'd drape them over the space heater in the kitchen to finish drying. One day she had her favorite red sweatshirt hanging over the space heater. Suddenly, the sleeve of the sweatshirt burst into flames!

Jean grabbed the sweatshirt by a corner that wasn't burning and threw it on the floor. She was going to stamp out the fire, but she wasn't wearing shoes. She didn't have a fire extinguisher in the kitchen. She grabbed a dirty pan full of water soaking in the sink and dumped it on the sweatshirt. That put out the fire. The kitchen floor was a mess of ashes and dirty water. Her favorite sweatshirt was ruined. But at least the fire was out and no one was hurt.

What did Jean do wrong? What did Jean do right? What could Jean have done differently?

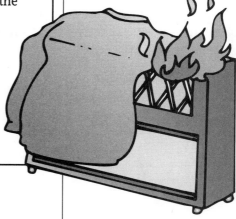

34

Preventing Fires: Flammable Products

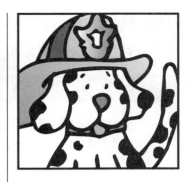

The Rule	The Reason
Never store flammable liquids near a heat source.	Gasoline, kerosene, charcoal lighter, and other liquids can start fires easily. Even one spark can cause a fire.

Introduction

When we think of liquids, we think of something that doesn't burn, like water. But some liquids do burn, like gasoline, kerosene, and charcoal lighter. Some paints and products containing alcohol also burn easily.

Activity

Write the word *FLAMMABLE* on the board in large letters. Explain that flammable means "likely to burn." Many flammable liquids, like gasoline, are kept in red containers. Bring an empty gas can to class to show the children.

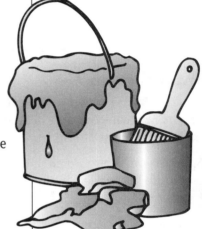

Some flammable products are not kept in red containers, however, and children should be aware of this. Rubbing alcohol, some hair sprays, and spray paints are commonly used products that are also flammable. Bring in several types of flammable products. Let children look for the warning labels.

Discussion

What are some examples of a heat source? (Fireplace, furnace, and heaters.) Why shouldn't you store flammable liquids near a heat source? Do all flammable liquids come in red cans?

Preventing Electrical Fires

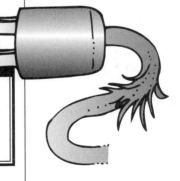

The Rule	The Reason
If you see any electrical cords that are worn or frayed, unplug them and tell an adult at once.	A broken electrical cord could easily start a fire.

Introduction

Electrical fires often occur due to overloaded outlets and broken or frayed electrical cords. More information about electrical safety can be found in Part 4: Household Safety.

Activity

Let children do a "cord check" in your classroom or another room in the school. Are there too many items plugged into one outlet? Are the cords worn or frayed? Ask children to do a "cord check" at home with their parents.

PREVENTING FIRES:
FIRECRACKERS, SPARKLERS, AND FIREWORKS

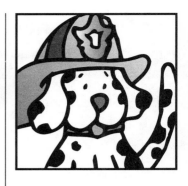

The Rules	The Reasons
Never play with sparklers or other types of fireworks unless an adult is present.	Even with an adult present, be very careful with sparklers. The tip of a lit sparkler is extremely hot. It can burn your hair or clothing. Hold the tip well away from yourself and other people.
Let an adult light the sparklers.	Do not play with matches.
Do not play with firecrackers.	In many places, firecrackers are illegal because so many people have been hurt by them.

Introduction

Firecrackers are explosives and very dangerous. If they explode near or close to your eyes or ears, you could become blind or deaf. They can burn you or blow off parts of your body. Firecrackers are NOT toys.

Sparklers are fun to watch, but they can be dangerous. When lit, a sparkler gets very hot. Never use lit sparklers in the house. You can have an adult place a lit candle in a sturdy holder on concrete and use that to light the sparklers.

Although legal, many types of fireworks are still dangerous and should be used with extreme caution. Even the legal kind must be lit, and anything that is lit could cause burns or start fires.

Warn children that many types of fireworks are not legal to have without a special license. Fireworks are neat to watch, but leave lighting them to the experts.

Discussion

What would you do if you found a package of firecrackers and some matches at the park? How could a lit sparkler start a fire? What would you do if a sparkler started your clothes on fire? (Stop! Drop! Roll!)

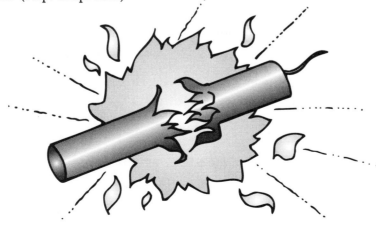

36

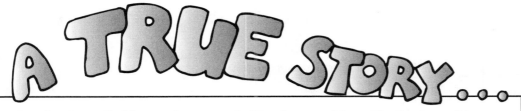

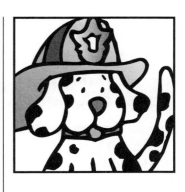

One day Jim called his mother at work. "Don't worry, Mom. The fire is out," he said.

"Fire! What fire?" she asked.

"The one on the garage roof," he told her.

"How did the garage roof start on fire?" she asked.

"My brother and I were playing with spinners and one landed on the garage roof. It got caught under the shingles and started the roof on fire." (Spinners are legal fireworks that jump into the air and spin when lit.)

"What did you do?" she asked.

"I yelled for help and my brother called the fire department. The neighbor lady heard me and came over with a fire extinguisher. She put out the fire before the fire trucks came."

"I'm glad no one was hurt and the garage wasn't burned down, but no more fireworks when I'm not home," she told him.

"OK, Mom. Bye."

What did Jim and his brother do wrong? What did they do right? What should they have done differently?

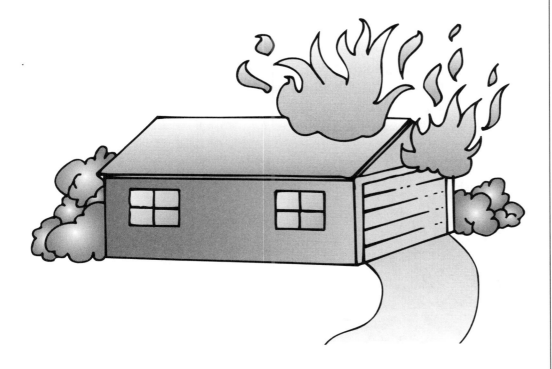

BUILDING FIRES SAFELY IN FIREPLACES AND WOOD-BURNING STOVES

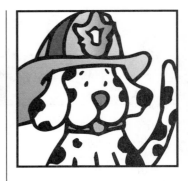

The Rules	The Reasons
If you have a fireplace or wood-burning stove, never start a fire by yourself.	Only adults should use matches and start fires. An adult should be present or nearby the entire time a fire is burning.
Use a metal screen in front of the fireplace.	A metal screen keeps sparks from jumping out and landing on you or the floor.
Make sure the fire is completely out before leaving the room.	It takes a long time for a fire to go out in a fireplace or wood-burning stove. The ashes can remain hot enough to start a fire for several hours.
Never use gasoline, lighter fluid, or charcoal lighter in a fireplace or wood-burning stove.	This could cause large flames and a fire that gets out of control.
Keep the wood inside the fireplace.	A piece of burning or hot wood could start a fire or burn you.
Don't store newspapers, matches, flammable liquids, or items that burn easily near a fireplace or wood-burning stove.	One spark could cause a fire to start outside the fireplace or wood-burning stove.
Use stones as a base at the bottom of the campfire.	This helps keep the fire in a small area.
Keep the fire small.	It is easier to control a small fire. With large fires, you will have more sparks flying. Flying sparks could land outside the camp area and start a forest fire.

BUILDING CAMPFIRES SAFELY

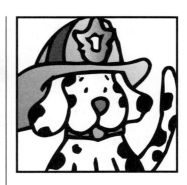

The Rules	The Reason
Don't get too close to a campfire.	Flying sparks could start your clothing on fire. If you cook hot dogs or marshmallows on sticks over the fire, be sure to use long sticks that won't burn.
Make sure the fire is completely out before leaving the area.	Even a few hot embers can blaze up and begin burning.
Start campfires only in designated areas.	In some areas, it is not safe to build a campfire.
Always let an adult start the fire.	Children should never start fires, even with an adult present.
Never pour gasoline or lighter fluid on a fire once it starts.	This could cause an explosion or an uncontrolled fire.

Introduction

Most people enjoy watching the flickering flames of a controlled fire in a fireplace or a campfire. Food cooked over a campfire seems to taste especially good. Almost everyone enjoys roasting marshmallows on sticks over a campfire or grill.

Children need to be aware that any fire can become dangerous if it gets out of control.

Activities

Have children review fire-safety rules by completing the reproducible on page 40, "You Can Prevent Fires."

Make copies of the parent letter on page 42 for children to take home and share with their parents.

Make a copy of the reproducible, "Fire Safety at the Browns," for each child. Let children complete the activity individually. When they finish, go through it with the class. Ask different children to tell which items they circled and why. If children missed some items, encourage them to circle them at that time.

Encourage children to make fire-safety posters and display them in the classroom. Have them make up fire-safety slogans and print them on their posters.

You Can Prevent Fires

Draw a picture to show each fire-safety rule.

Keep campfires small.	Stop! Drop! Roll!
If a door is closed and you smell smoke, don't open the door.	Go to a neighbor's to call for help if there is a fire in your house.
Know two exits from each room in your house.	Never store flammable liquids near a heat source.

Fire Safety at the Brown's

The Brown family is prepared for fire safety. Circle all the fire-safety precautions you can find in the picture. Color the picture.

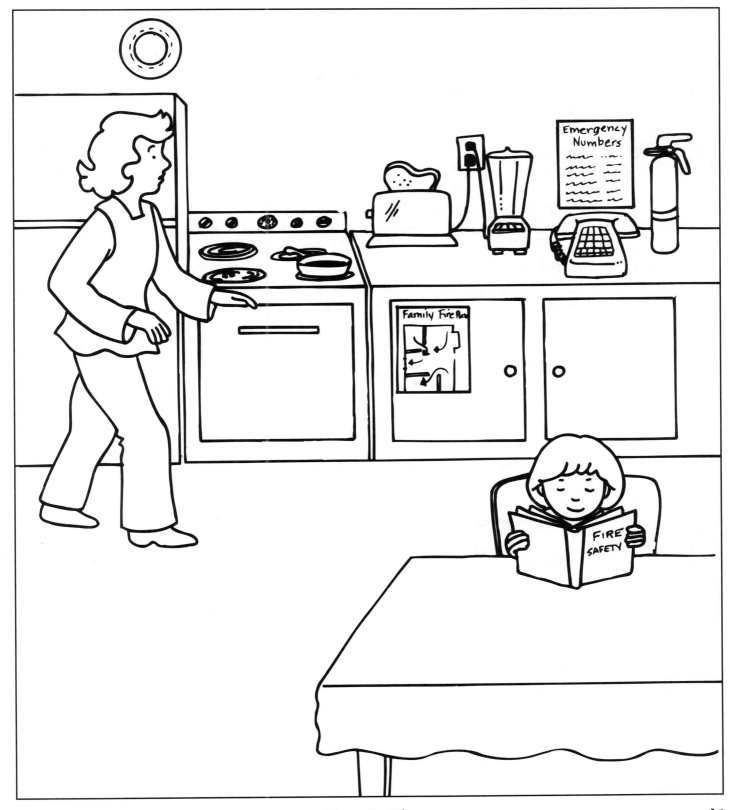

Dear Parents,

We have been studying about fire safety in class. We have learned about smoke detectors, fire extinguishers, and fire drills. We practiced Stop! Drop! Roll! Here are reminders about fire safety in your home. Please review fire safety with your children so they know what to do if a fire starts. Remind them of the importance of remaining calm and acting quickly.

Fire Extinguishers

● Do you have fire extinguishers in your home? Fire extinguishers should be in your kitchen, garage, and basement. Show your children where the fire extinguishers are kept and how to use them. If a small fire can be put out quickly, do so. If not, get out at once and call for help. A small fire can easily turn into a big fire.

Smoke Detectors

● Do you have smoke detectors on every level of your home and in the garage?
● Do you check your smoke detectors monthly to make sure the batteries aren't dead? If you haven't checked them lately, today is a good time to start.

Family Fire Plan and Drills

● You and your family should have a fire plan. A fire plan lets everyone know what to do and where to go if a fire starts in your house.
● Practice your plan. Teach children two exits from every room, including the basement. Hold family fire drills.
● Have a planned meeting place outside for your family. You'll know quickly if anyone is missing.
● If you live in an apartment, remind children not to use the elevators during a fire. Make certain everyone in the family knows where the stairways and fire exits are located.

Fire Prevention

● Keep matches and lighters away from children.
● Remind children never to light a candle or to make a fire in the fireplace or wood-burning stove without your approval.
● Store flammable liquids away from heat sources.
● Check electrical cords. Get rid of any that are worn or frayed.
● Do not overload outlets.
● Do not run electrical cords under carpets or rugs.

Household Safety

Kitchen Safety

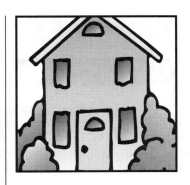

The Rules	The Reasons
Wipe up spills on the floor right away.	Someone might slip and fall.
Watch out for sharp edges on can covers.	You could get a bad cut.
Plastic bags are not toys. Do not play with them or put them over your head.	You will not be able to breathe.
Chew well before swallowing.	You could choke.
Don't gulp your food.	Taste food carefully to make sure it isn't too hot. Food in a microwave cooks from the inside out. Even if the outside doesn't feel very hot, the inside could be much hotter.
Don't lean back too far on your chair.	You could tip over.
When you play Hide and Seek, never hide in a stove, refrigerator, freezer, or other place where you may get trapped.	Many appliances cannot be opened from the inside. You could be trapped and not have enough air to breathe.

Introduction

The kitchen is typically the most dangerous room in a house. Cuts, burns, slips, and falls are among the more common injuries that occur. Children are taught to Stop! Look! and Listen! when crossing streets. In the kitchen, the motto could be "Stop! Think! Do!"

Discussion

What do you think "Stop! Think! Do!" means? Can you give some examples where this would be a good motto? What would you do if you saw your little brother or sister playing with a plastic bag? Should you take it away even if it makes the child cry? Why? Which of the safety rules above do you think is the most important? Why?

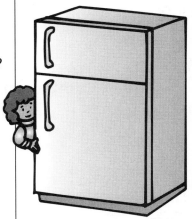

KITCHEN SAFETY: OVENS AND MICROWAVES

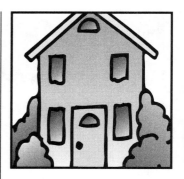

The Rules	The Reasons
Do not touch a hot stove.	Hot stoves can cause burns.
Always turn the handles of pans on the stove towards the back.	If handles are hanging over the front edge of the stove, someone may knock the pans over and spill the hot food. This could cause a serious burn.

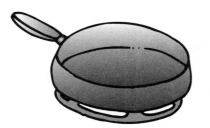

Never operate a stove or microwave without permission.	If you do any cooking on a stove or microwave, it is best to have an adult present.
A bowl or cup can become very hot when heated in a microwave.	Always use oven mitts when removing anything from the microwave.
Never try to cook a new type of food until you read the directions carefully.	Some foods, like potatoes and hot dogs, can explode if the skin isn't pricked before cooking. Other foods trap hot steam which can shoot out and burn you when you take them from the microwave.
After taking food from the microwave, open containers away from yourself and other people.	Hot steam may be trapped inside a container. Open bags, covers, and plastic wrap carefully to avoid burning yourself or other people.

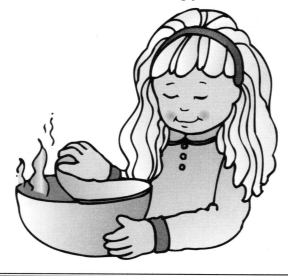

44

The Rules	The Reasons
Never put any metal object in a microwave. Silverware, cups, or dishes with metal trim should not be used.	Metal objects in a microwave will start a fire. Even the small amount of metal in a twist tie can cause a fire.

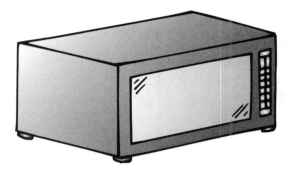 

Never turn on a microwave when it is empty.	This can damage the microwave.

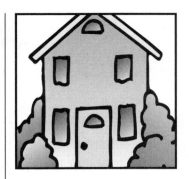

Introduction

Ovens and microwaves are conveniences many of would find it difficult to do without. Unfortunately, these appliances can be major hazards to children and adults. Burns from hot pans, dishes, and steam are painful. A burn caused by spilling hot grease or hot liquid can be extremely painful and serious. By learning to use ovens and microwaves safely and being aware of potential dangers, children and adults can reduce the risk of injury to themselves and others in the kitchen.

Discussion

Make a copy of "Kitchen Safety: Ovens and Microwaves Rules and Reasons" on page 44 for each child. Go through each safety rule and reason as children follow along. Stop and let children talk about specific instances of kitchen safety. Invite children to take home their copies to share with their parents.

Do you help your parents make meals? What do you like to make?

What would you do if you saw your younger brother or sister playing with the knobs on the stove? What would you do if you saw your younger brother or sister climb up on a chair and push the buttons on the microwave?

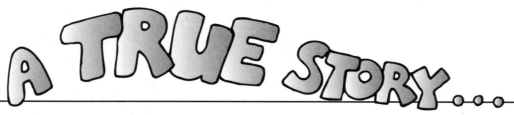

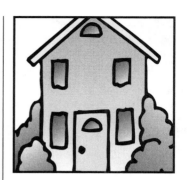

Tom decided to defrost a bagel in the microwave. He wrapped it in a napkin and put it on a paper plate. He put it in the microwave and set the timer for 30 seconds. He stood by the microwave while it was cooking. With only eight seconds left on the timer, Tom suddenly saw flames in the microwave. He opened the door, grabbed the plate by one corner, and dumped the whole thing in the dish pan in the kitchen sink. The napkin, paper plate, and bagel were all partly burned. Then he discovered that the twist tie from the bagel package had fallen on the plate before he put it into the microwave. That's what started the fire.

What did Tom do wrong? What did he do right? What could he have done differently?

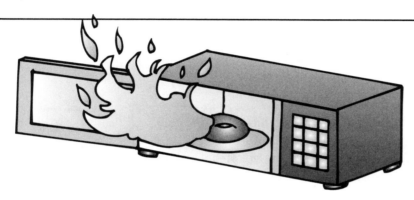

Activities

Bring in several twist ties from bread wrappers. Let children peel off the paper to reveal the metal wire inside. Bring some other ceramic cups or bowls with metal trim as examples of the type of containers that cannot be used in a microwave. Also bring in containers that are safe to use in a microwave.

Take children to the school cafeteria kitchen, and ask one of the workers to demonstrate several kitchen-safety rules children have learned. This works best if you and the kitchen worker plan in advance.

Set up a demonstration kitchen in your classroom. Use a large upside-down cardboard box, for a pretend stove. Draw burners on it with black marker. Use another smaller box for a microwave. A third box can serve as a kitchen cupboard. Bring in some real pans and utensils. (If you don't have spares, pick up some inexpensive ones at a rummage sale or flea market.)

Let children make other items you need for your classroom kitchen, like a smoke detector (from a large plastic lid) and a fire extinguisher from an empty two-liter plastic soda bottle wrapped in red construction paper. Let children practice kitchen safety in their demo kitchen by preparing pretend meals.

Natural Gas

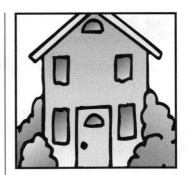

The Rules	The Reasons
If you turn on a gas stove or other gas appliance and the flame does not appear in about five seconds, turn it off.	The gas could build up and explode.
Notify an adult immediately if you smell gas.	If you are home alone and smell gas, leave immediately. Do not light a match or turn on a light switch. Do not use the telephone. This could cause a spark and the gas could explode. Go to a neighbor's house and call for help.

Introduction

Many appliances, like stoves, water heaters, dryers, and furnaces use natural gas. Natural gas itself is odorless. A chemical is added to natural gas so that the smell is easily recognized.

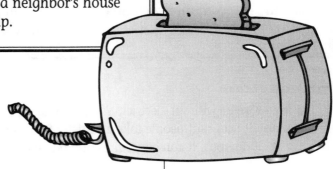

Activity

Contact your local power company and ask if they have any "scratch and sniff" samples that you can bring to your class. Let children scratch and sniff. Once they smell the distinctive odor of the chemical added to natural gas, they will probably recognize it immediately if a gas leak ever develops.

Electrical Safety

The Rules	The Reasons
Never stick a metal object, like a knife, in a toaster when it is plugged in.	You could get an electrical shock. If a piece of bread, English muffin, or bagel gets stuck in the toaster, unplug it. Wait until the toaster cools before trying to get it out.
Never use an electrical appliance like a radio or hair dryer in or near water.	Water and electricity do not go together. If the appliance falls in water, you could get an electrical shock.
Do not plug in a cord with wet hands or while standing on a wet floor.	You could get an electrical shock.

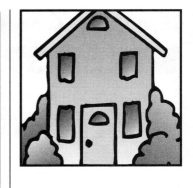

The Rules	The Reasons
Don't touch electrical outlets with your fingers or with anything else.	You could get an electrical shock.
Remove electrical cords from the outlet by pulling on the plug, not the cord.	Pulling on the cord can damage it. Broken or frayed cords can cause fires.
Do not stretch electrical cords across the room.	Someone might trip on them.
Do not run electrical cords under a carpet or rug.	The cords could get worn, broken, or frayed. Cords that are broken, worn, or frayed could cause a fire.
Plug only one cord into each hole of an outlet.	Fires can be caused by plugging too many electrical cords into one outlet.

Introduction

Where would we be without electricity? We depend on so many different types of electrical appliances that people take electricity for granted. They forget that electricity can also be dangerous. It can cause fires and bad electrical shocks.

Discussion

What are some electrical appliances you have at your house? What do you think it would be life if we didn't have electricity? Could people cook without electricity? How? Could people have light and heat without electricity? How? What are some things you enjoy doing that you could not do without electricity?

Activities

Demonstrate how to correctly unplug appliances by pulling on the plug, not the cord.

Ask children to make Electrical Safety posters to display in your classroom.

Children may not realize how much we rely on electrical appliances or how many appliances need electricity to operate. Have children cut out pictures of many different types of electrical appliances from old magazine or catalogs and glue them to a large piece of posterboard.

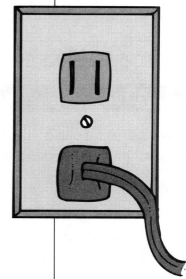

Contact your local power/electric company. Ask if they have a speaker available to talk about electrical safety with your class. Encourage children to ask questions and participate in the discussion. If the power/electric company does not have a speaker available, find out if they have electrical safety posters or other related materials that can be used in your classroom.

Bathroom Safety

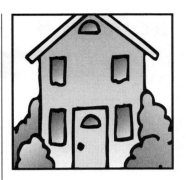

The Rules	The Reasons
Never play with the faucets in the shower or tub.	You could accidentally turn on the hot water and get burned.
Use a rubber mat in the tub or shower.	This will help prevent falls in slippery tubs and showers.
Keep the floor by the shower or tub dry.	It can be slippery when wet!
Keep all medicines out of the reach of children.	Many medicines are dangerous if taken by the wrong person. See the section on "Poisons and Other Hazardous Household Products" on pages 51–52.

Slips, Trips, and Falls

The Rules	The Reasons
If something spills, wipe it up right away.	Someone could slip and fall. Wet floors are slippery.
Keep toys picked up and put away.	Someone could trip over them and fall. Falls hurt.
Always put tools back where they belong.	Someone could trip over them and fall.
Don't carry anything so large you can't see over it.	If you try to carry a large pile and can't see over the top, you may trip and fall.
Don't climb on unstable objects to reach items.	Chairs, crates and drawers are NOT safe to climb on. Use a ladder or ask an adult to help you reach something on a high shelf.
Keep stairs clear of toys and other obstacles.	Someone might trip and fall.
Never jump on beds and furniture.	You might fall and hit your head.

Discussion

Ask children to give reasons for each of these rules.

- Stairs are for walking, not playing.
- Walk, don't run, up and down the steps.
- Use handrails on stairs.
- Don't slide or walk on the railings.

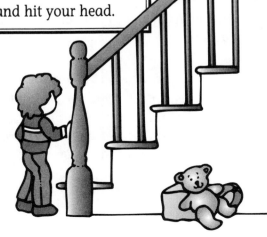

Bedroom Safety

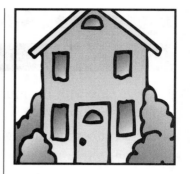

The Rules	The Reasons
Never check out strange sounds by yourself.	If you hear sounds at night, call an adult to check it out.
Keep a night-light burning or turn on a light when you walk around at night.	You won't trip over objects in the dark or run into furniture.
Don't jump on the bed.	Beds are for sleeping. If you jump on them, you might fall and get hurt.

Introduction

Many children enjoy playing in their bedrooms. Some activities, like board games, coloring, and reading are fine. Other games that are more active, like tag and jumping contests, should be held outside.

Discussion

Why do you think it would be a good idea to call an adult if you hear a strange sound at night?

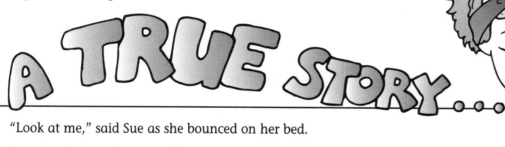

A True Story...

"Look at me," said Sue as she bounced on her bed.

"I can go higher than that," her sister, Sara, answered. "Watch me!" Sara jumped higher. When she landed, she hit her head on the edge of the headboard and cut her forehead.

Do you think that was a good contest? Was Sara the winner? Where would be a safe place for Sara and Sue to have a jumping contest?

Activities

Remind children that jumping on beds and furniture could cause injuries by singing this song with them about the five little monkeys.

Five Little Monkeys

Five little monkeys, jumping on the bed.
One fell off and bumped his head.
Mama called the doctor. The doctor said,
"No more monkey business on that bed."

Repeat with four, three, two and one monkey.

Poisons and Other Hazardous Household Products

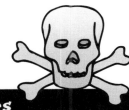

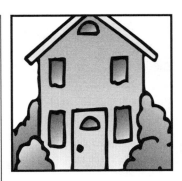

The Rules	The Reasons
Never eat, drink, or even open products unless you know what they are and how to use them.	Even things that smell or taste good may be poison. Many types of cleaners have a pleasant smell, but don't be fooled.

Introduction

Many liquids and powders used around the house, garage, and yard are useful and necessary, but they can make you sick if you eat or drink them. Some products used around the house can damage your eyes or skin.

Many types of cleaners have a pleasant smell, but don't be fooled. Just because something smells good doesn't mean it's good to eat or drink. Some dangerous products have a symbol that looks like a skull, but not all dangerous products are labeled.

Discussion

Discuss the meaning of the words *poisonous* and *hazardous*. Ask children to name different types of products that could make them sick or cause injury to their eyes or skin. (Insecticides, weed killers, medicines, cleaning supplies, oven cleaners, furniture polish, bleach, ammonia, laundry detergent, lighter fluid, gasoline, kerosene, paint, and paint thinner are a few examples.)

Where does your family keep these kinds of dangerous products?

Are they on a high shelf? Are they in a locked cabinet? Ask your parents to put poisons on a high shelf or in a locked cabinet so your younger brothers and sisters will be safe, too.

Medicines

The Rules	The Reasons
Never take any medicine unless it is given to you by a responsible adult.	Medicine from a doctor should only be taken by the person it was prescribed for. Even over-the-counter medicines can be dangerous or make you sick if taken incorrectly.

Introduction

Other hazardous products kept around the house are prescription and over-the-counter medicines. Medicines are good. They help us get well, but they can be very dangerous too. Some pills look like candy, but they aren't. They are medicine. Medicine can make you well, but it can also make you sick if not taken by the right person in the right way.

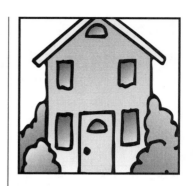

Discussion

If you find a bottle of pills that look like candy, what should you do? Why do you think medicines like cough syrup are made to taste good? Should you use cherry cough syrup as a topping on your ice cream? Where should medicines be kept? When should you take medicine? Are all the medicines in your house kept in one place, high enough that little children cannot reach them?

Activity

Let children make their own warning labels. Get a sheet of brightly-colored round labels for each child. Let children decorate the labels with yucky faces using pens or markers. They can take the labels home and, with an adult, put the labels on hazardous products. This will help the child and the entire family become more aware of what hazardous products are in the house and where they are kept.

SPRAY CANS

The Rules	The Reasons
Do not play with spray cans. Never spray anything near anyone's eyes, nose, or mouth.	Spray cans can be dangerous. They may contain products that are hazardous. Some sprays can damage eyes or skin.
Never put a spray can in a fire.	Spray cans can explode if they become too hot.

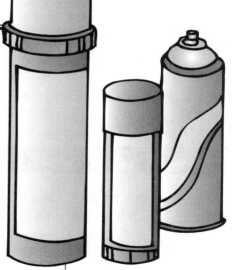

Introduction

Many products in spray cans can be dangerous. Even a common item like hair spray can cause injury to the eyes.

Discussion

What types of products in spray cans do you have at your house?

Activity

Bring several different types of empty spray cans to class. Explain the words *toxic* and *flammable*. Read the warning labels on the cans with children. Ask them to explain what the warnings mean in their own words.

PLANTS

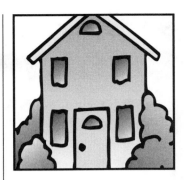

The Rules	The Reasons
Never eat any part of a plant unless you know it's safe. This includes flowers, leaves, berries, fruits, nuts, and mushrooms.	Some common household and garden plants are poisonous.
Wash all raw fruits and vegetables before eating them.	Some fruits and vegetables are sprayed with insect or weed killers. These chemicals can make you sick.

Discussion

What would you do if you saw your baby brother or sister chewing on the leaves of a plant at your house?

What if your friend picked some berries off a bush while you were walking home from school? "Try these," your friend says. "They're good."

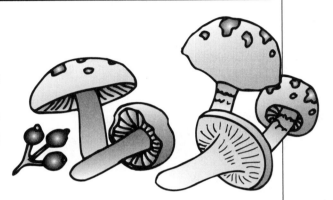

You don't know what kind of berries they are. What should you do?

Activity

Ask children to draw pictures of a family following safety rules about poisons and other hazardous household products.

WEAPONS

The Rules	The Reasons
Guns and other weapons should be locked away at all times.	Weapons are very dangerous. You could injure yourself or someone else.

What to Do

If you see a gun, do not play with it. It is not a toy. Even if you are sure it is not loaded, do not touch it. Call an adult to put it away in a safe, locked place.

Safety with Sharp Objects

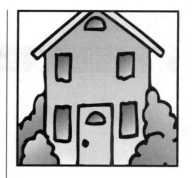

The Rules	The Reasons
Never use sharp objects or tools with sharp edges without an adult's permission.	Objects like knives, saws, axes, and screwdrivers can cause bad cuts if not used correctly and carefully.
Put the item away as soon as you finish using it.	A younger child might pick up the sharp object and get hurt. If left on the floor or the ground, someone might step on it.
Store tools with sharp edges so the sharp edge is turned away.	This will prevent someone from getting cut when he or she reaches for the item.

Discussion

What are some examples of sharp objects that could cut you?

Activities

Make a copy of the reproducible "The Safe Way" on page 56 for each child. Have children complete the activity independently. When they finish, go through the activity with the class and ask different children to tell which pictures they circled. If someone missed a picture or circled the wrong one, let them correct it with the class.

Play Household Safety Concentration. Photocopy pages 57 and 58 on heavy paper or light cardboard. Make several sets so children can play in small groups. Cut out the cards and mix them up. Place the cards in rows, face down. You may want to use only five or six sets of cards for very young children.

The first child turns over two cards. If the cards match, the child keeps the cards and turns over two more. If the cards do not match, the child turns the cards back face down and play continues with the next child. The game ends when all pairs are matched. Shuffle the cards and play again.

If you have the resources, make one set of cards for each child in the class to take home and play with their families.

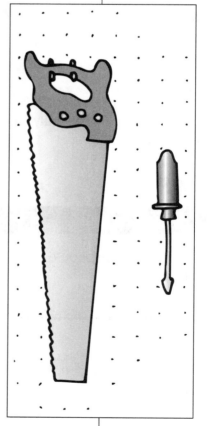

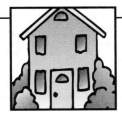

Dear Parents,

We have been studying about home safety in class. Your child has learned about many possible safety hazards in the home and what to do about them. Would you take a few minutes to go through this home safety inspection checklist with your child? If you find a problem, correct it as soon as possible, for safety's sake.

Kitchen

_____ Do you remember to turn the handles of pots and pans on the stove towards the back?

_____ Are plastic bags stored out of reach of young children?

_____ Have children been taught when and how to use the stove and microwave safely?

_____ Do you set a good example by wiping up spills as soon as they happen so no one slips and falls?

Bathroom

_____ Do you have non-slip mats in the bathtub and shower?

_____ Are all medicines kept in a high place, out of reach of children?

Bedrooms

_____ Do you have nightlights in the bedrooms and hallways so no one will stumble on objects on the floor if they get up at night?

Basement and Garage

_____ Have the doors been removed from discarded appliances?

_____ Are weed killers, insecticides, and other hazardous products kept on a high shelf or locked cabinet out of reach of children?

_____ Are sharp tools stored out of reach of children?

Stairs

_____ Are stairways kept free of objects that could cause someone to trip and fall?

_____ Are railings loose?

Climbing

_____ Do you set a good example by climbing on a step stool or ladder when you need to reach something on a high shelf?

Electrical

_____ Do any of your power tools or appliances have frayed or worn cords?

_____ Have children been taught not to use power tools without direct supervision?

_____ Are there too many cords plugged into one outlet?

_____ Are any electrical cords under rugs or carpeting?

_____ Are any electrical cords near heat-producing appliances?

_____ Are all small electrical appliances kept far from sinks and tubs?

Weapons

_____ Do you keep all guns, arrows, hunting knives, and other potential weapons in a locked place?

THE SAFE WAY

Look at the pictures in each box. Circle the pictures that demonstrate safety rules.

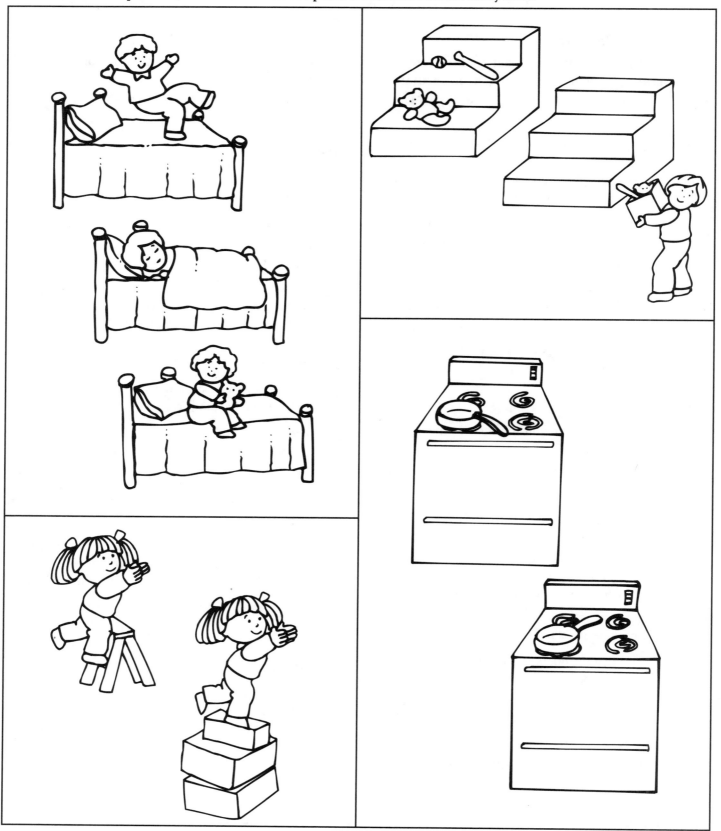

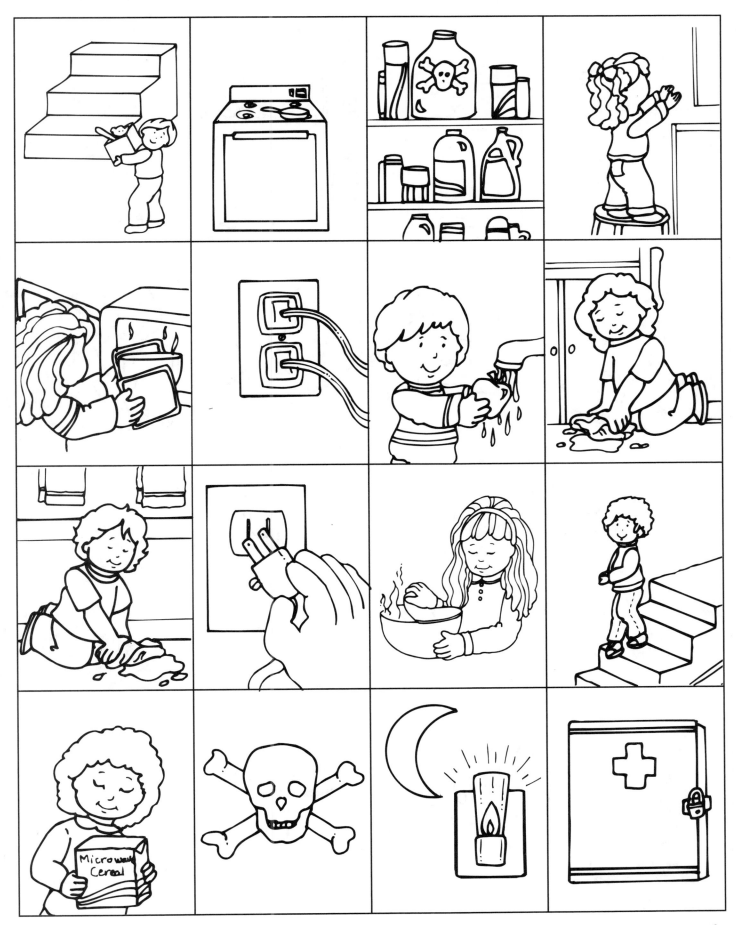

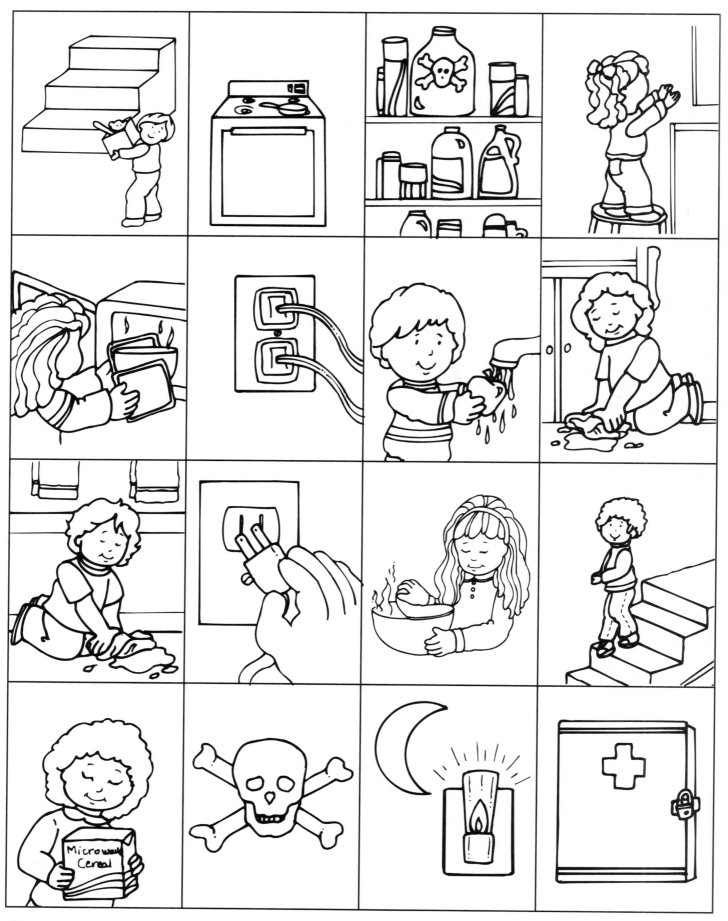

Sports Safety

Safe Bicycle Riding

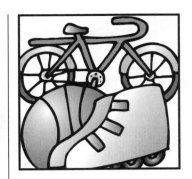

The Rules	The Reasons

Use reflectors and lights when riding at night. Wear light-colored clothing.

It is easier for drivers to see you.

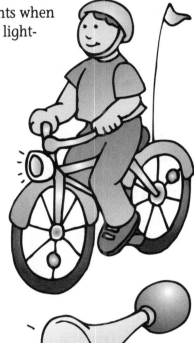

Don't show off.

Trick riding is for circus clowns. You could fall and get hurt.

Warn others when you approach by sounding your horn or bell. If you don't have one, call out.

Running into someone could hurt both of you.

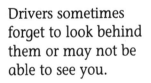

Watch for cars backing out of driveways.

Drivers sometimes forget to look behind them or may not be able to see you.

Keep both hands on the handle bars.

You may loose your balance and fall if you ride one-handed.

Always wear a helmet when you ride your bicycle.

If you fall, a helmet will protect your head.

The Rules	The Reasons

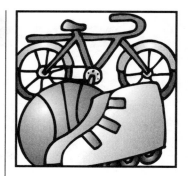

Never hang on to the back of a moving vehicle when riding your bike.

You may lose your balance and fall.

Don't ride a bike that's too big for you.

If the bike is too big, you may not be able to control it or stop safely. You may lose your balance and fall.

Don't ride double or carry packages on your handlebars that are too high to see over the top. Carry packages in a basket.

The rider may not be able to see where he or she is going.

Ride single file. Don't ride in the middle of the street. Stay on the right side of the street, along the curb.

Always ride in the same direction as traffic. You may be hit by a car if you are in the middle of the street.

Don't hold hands with another bicycle rider.

You may both lose your balance and fall.

Watch for hazards in the road like bumps, obstacles, and railroad tracks.

They could cause you to lose control of your bike and fall.

Always pay attention to where you are going.

Looking backwards could cause you to ride into a parked car.

60

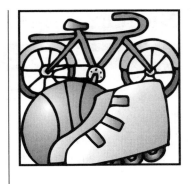

Introduction

Knowing safe bicycle-riding rules and following them will keep you and others safe.

Discussion

Make copies of the "Safe Bicycle Riding Rules and Reasons" on pages 59 and 60 for each child. Read through the rules and reasons as children follow along. Periodically stop and ask children what they would do if they saw one of their friends breaking the discussed safety rule.

Encourage children to take their copies of "Safe Bicycle Rules and Reasons" home and discuss scenarios with their families.

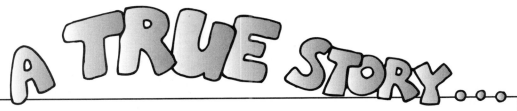

Jay was riding his bike to a friend's house one evening. It was dark out, but Jay wore a light-colored jacket. His bike had reflectors and a light. Jay was thinking about the video games he and his friend were going to play. Suddenly, Jay found himself flying through the air, over the top of a parked car. He landed in the street with a broken leg.

What did Jay do right? What did Jay do wrong? What could he have done to avoid breaking his leg?

Activities

Ask children to draw pictures of themselves following one of the bicycle safety rules.

Ask a police officer to speak to your class about bicycle safety. Encourage children to ask questions and participate in the discussion.

Set up cones and cardboard boxes for a bicycle obstacle course on the playground. Let children practice riding through the course safely. Do not emphasize speed in completing the course.

Invite a bicycle repair specialist or one of the student's parents, to demonstrate checking items on the bicycle maintenance list. If possible, have a bicycle that needs some minor repairs and fix it during the demonstration. Encourage children to participate.

Hold a bicycle safety roundup. Have several adults with tools available to help children check their bicycles and complete minor repairs.

Does your city require bicycle licenses? Find out how and where to obtain them in your community. Check which children in the class do not have a bike license and help them obtain one.

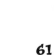

Bicycle Traffic Rules

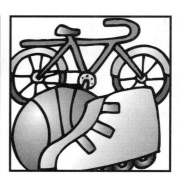

The Rules	The Reasons

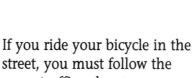

Stop at all stop signs. Check for traffic before you go.

Stop at all stoplights if the light is yellow or red. Go only on a green light.

Stop at all flashing red lights. Slow down and be cautious if you see a flashing yellow light.

When stopped at a corner, watch for cars making right turns.

If you must make a left turn and there is a lot of traffic, get off your bike and walk it across the street when the light is green.

Always signal when making a turn.

If you ride your bicycle in the street, you must follow the same traffic rules as cars, buses, and motorcycles.

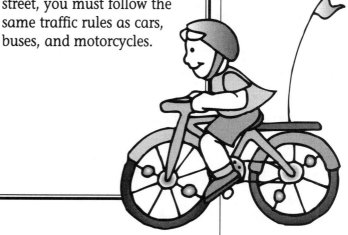

Introduction

Traffic rules help keep everyone on the road safe—bicycle riders; drivers of cars, buses, and motorcycles; and people walking.

Discussion

Why is it important to understand and obey traffic signs when riding your bike? How is riding a bike in the street like driving a car?

Activities

Post a copy of the "Safe Bicycle Riding" and "Bicycle Traffic Rules and Reasons" in your classroom to remind children throughout the year.

Make a copy of the activity sheet, "Catch Them Doing Something Right!"on page 64 for each child. Invite children to complete the activity individually. Then go through it with the class, asking different children to tell which items they circled and why. If children missed some items, encourage them to circle them at that time.

Make copies and distribute the activity sheet, "Traffic Signs and Hand Signals You Should Know" on page 63. Let children discuss what each sign means and how it affects them when they are riding their bikes.

Demonstrate the proper hand signals for a left turn, right turn, and stop. Have children practice these hand signals as they take a pretend ride around the playground.

TRAFFIC SIGNS AND HAND SIGNALS YOU SHOULD KNOW

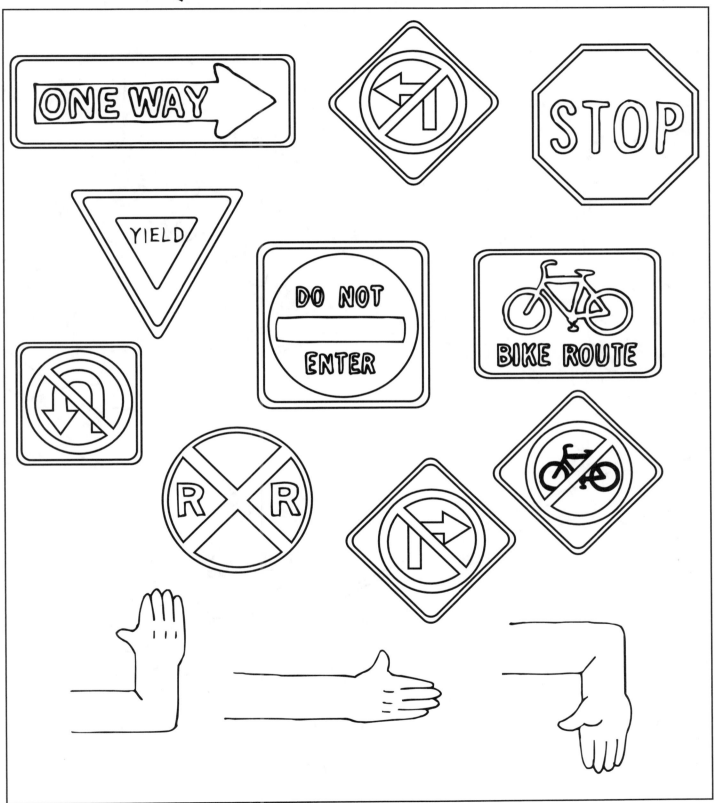

CATCH THEM DOING SOMETHING RIGHT!

Study the picture below. Circle all the parts of the picture that show safe bicycle riding, like children wearing helmets.

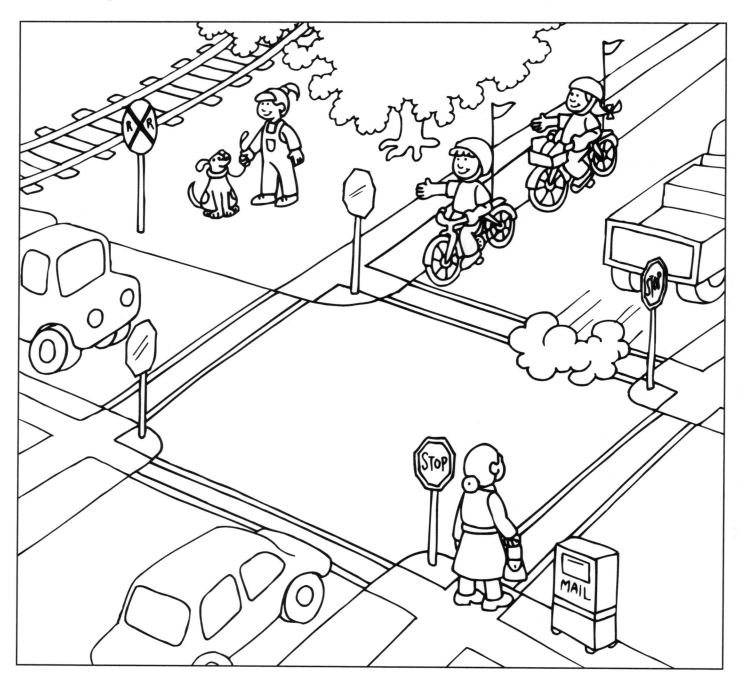

What bicycle safety rule do you think is most important? Write your answer below.

_____

_____

Safe Bicycle Maintenance

If you are old enough to ride a bicycle, you are old enough to check that your bike is working properly. Riding a bike that needs repair can be dangerous. Some problems need to be fixed at a bicycle repair shop, others can be done by an adult at home. Keep this checklist handy and use it to inspect your bike for problems every week or two. If your bike needs repair, don't ride it until it can be fixed.

Bicycle Inspection Checklist

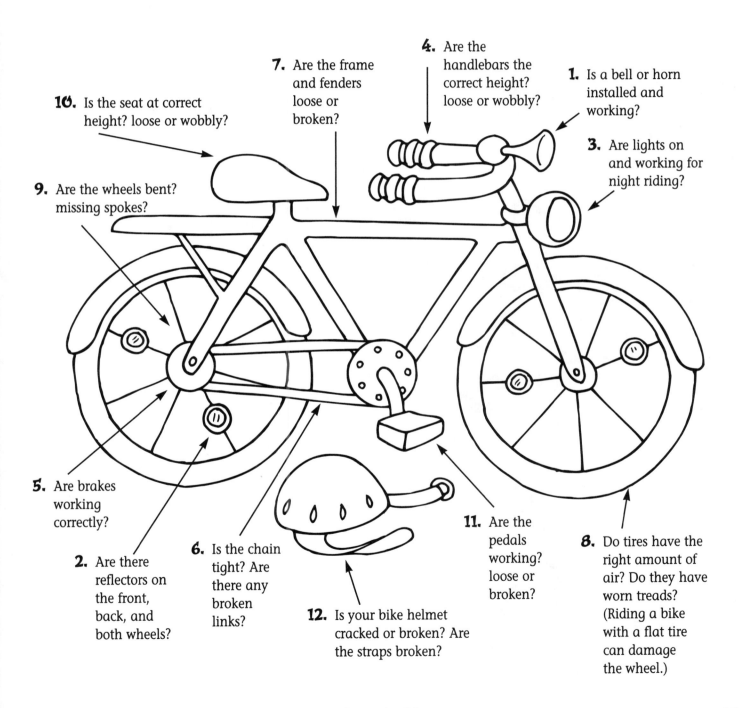

10. Is the seat at correct height? loose or wobbly?

7. Are the frame and fenders loose or broken?

4. Are the handlebars the correct height? loose or wobbly?

1. Is a bell or horn installed and working?

3. Are lights on and working for night riding?

9. Are the wheels bent? missing spokes?

5. Are brakes working correctly?

2. Are there reflectors on the front, back, and both wheels?

6. Is the chain tight? Are there any broken links?

12. Is your bike helmet cracked or broken? Are the straps broken?

11. Are the pedals working? loose or broken?

8. Do tires have the right amount of air? Do they have worn treads? (Riding a bike with a flat tire can damage the wheel.)

Reproducible

In-Line Skating and Skateboarding

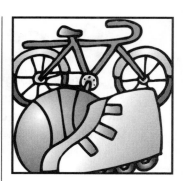

The Rules	The Reasons
Wear safety equipment.	Knee pads, elbow pads, wrist guards, and a helmet provide protection when skating and skateboarding. Gloves protect your hands against scrapes and cuts.

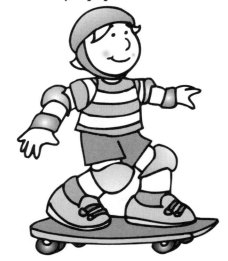

Skaters who play street hockey will need extra protection, including shin pads, hip pads, and a face-screened helmet.

Check your equipment.

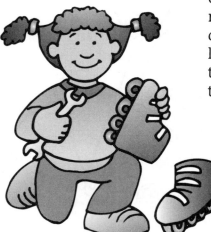

Each time you use your skateboard or in-line skates, check to see that all nuts, bolts, and screws are tight. Ask and adult to help you tighten any loose ones. Make sure the wheels turn freely and there are no cracks in the skateboard.

Skate in a safe place.

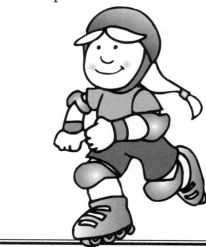

If you are going to skate or use your skateboard on the sidewalk, do it where there are not many people walking or younger children playing.

The Rules	The Reasons
Watch for obstacles. 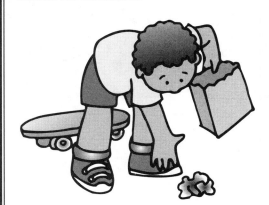	Check the area for litter, stones, and other items in the area where you plan to skate or skateboard. These items could cause you to fall. Clean up the area before you begin.
Follow the rules for street skating and skateboarding.	Some cities do not allow skaters or skateboarding on public streets. Find out what the rules are in your city. Your local police station can tell you.
Stay alert. 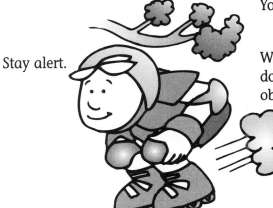	Watch where you are going so you don't run into anyone or trip over obstacles.
Be courteous.	Yield the right of way to people walking and children playing.

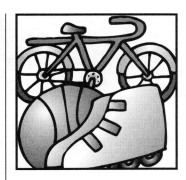

Introduction

The days when kids strapped on a pair of roller skates, tightened them with a skate key, and took off down the sidewalk seem to be a thing of the past. Today's in-line skates are faster, fancier, and much more expensive. What hasn't changed is that children still fall down while skating. They scrape their elbows and knees, and occasionally break an arm or leg. Wearing the variety of safety equipment available can reduce injuries.

Discussion

Make copies and distribute the "In-line Skating and Skateboarding Rules and Reasons" on pages 66 and 67. Read through the rules and reasons as children follow along.

How do knee pads and elbow pads protect you when skating or skateboarding? Why is it smart to wear a helmet? What does the phrase *Skate smart* mean to you?

Activities

Call your local police department and find out what the local regulations are for skating and skateboarding in the street. Relay this information to students.

Invite someone from a local sports shop to talk about safe skating and skateboarding, skating and skateboarding safety equipment, and skate and skateboard maintenance. If possible, ask the person to give a hands-on demonstration. Encourage children to ask questions and participate in the discussion.

Make a copy of the reproducible, "Skating Smart" on page 69 for each child. Read the rule in each box. Ask children to write or draw the reason for each rule.

Have children review the rules about wearing safety equipment as they complete the activity sheet, "Helping Children Play Safely" on page 70.

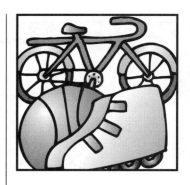

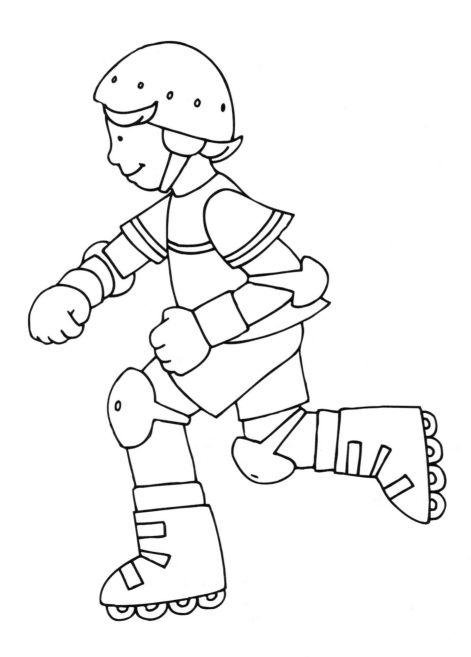

68

Skating Smart

Write or draw the reason for each skating and skateboarding rule.

Skate on the right side of the street or sidewalk.

Control your speed.

Stay off streets with heavy traffic.

Yield to pedestrians. Warn others when you are about to pass them.

Learn the basic skills of balance, stopping, turning, and falling safely in a safe, flat place before you try fancy tricks or skating on hills.

If you skate in the street, obey all traffic signs and traffic rules.

Helping Children Play Safely

These children want to have fun, but they have forgotten their safety equipment. Draw what they need to play safety.

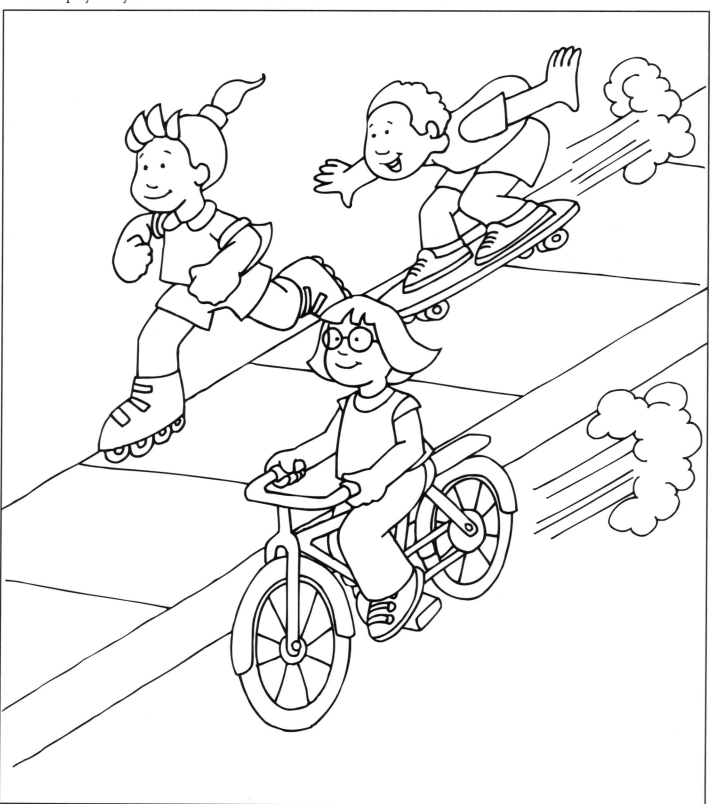

Kite-Flying Safety

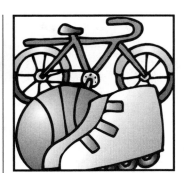

The Rules	The Reasons
Never fly a kite in a thunderstorm.	Lightning can be attracted to the kite, passing electricity down through the wet string to you.
Never use metal when building a kite.	Metal can attract lightning even if it isn't storming.
Wear gloves while flying a kite.	A fast-moving string can cut the skin on your hand.
Never fly a kite near telephone poles or power lines.	If a kite touches power lines, the electricity can travel down the string to you.
If a kite lands on or near wires, don't try to get it yourself.	Electricity can injure or kill. Call the police or fire department.
Don't fly your kite near trees. If your kite gets caught in a tree, let an adult help get it out.	Falling from a tree could be worse than losing your kite.
Don't walk across the street while flying a kite.	Your attention might be on the kite, not traffic.
Don't run across a street chasing a kite.	*Stop! Look* both ways! *Listen* before you cross a street. It is better to lose a kite than to get hit by a car.
It is against the law to fly a kite within five miles of any airport.	The kite or string could get caught in a plane's propeller.
Don't fly a kite near a cliff or steep drop-off.	You might fall off the edge. While you're looking up, you could fall down.

Introduction

Flying a kite on a brisk windy day can be great fun. Brightly-colored kites soaring across a blue sky are a beautiful sight. By following safety rules for kite-flying, everyone can have a fun and safe experience.

Discussion

Have you ever flown a kite? Which kite safety rule do you think is the most important? Why?

What happens when you fly a kite on a day when there isn't any wind? Why? What happens when you fly a kite on a day when it is too windy? Why?

A TRUE STORY...

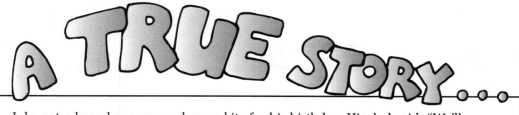

Jake got a brand-new super dragon kite for his birthday. His dad said, "We'll go kite-flying in the big field by the high school tomorrow when I get home from work if the weather is good. There aren't any trees or power lines close by."

But Jake was too excited to wait. It was a perfect kite-flying day, with just the right amount of wind. Before his dad got home from work, Jake took his kite out in the backyard and started to fly it. A gust of wind came up and blew his kite into a tree. Jake climbed the tree to get his kite. He lost his balance and fell out of the tree. He sprained his wrist. The kite was still stuck in the tree.

What did Jake do wrong? What should he have done? What happened to Jake? Why do you think it happened? What would you have done if you were Jake?

Activities

Let children make paper kites to decorate your classroom. Pre-cut white construction paper into diamond shapes, or the shapes of objects, like a large fish, hot-air balloon, or dragon. Let children decorate the kites with paint, crayons, and markers. Use tape to add a long, colorful tail of yarn or ribbon. Hang the kites on a wall in your classroom near the ceiling.

Write some safe kite-flying safety tips on banners to use as the tails of the kites.

Tie this section in with a unit on seasons. It is particularly relevant to a unit on spring or fall.

Children can make their own kites from medium-sized plastic bags with handles (the kind you get at most department stores). Give each child one bag and about 12 feet of kite string. Have them tie the handles together, but leave the bag open, so air blows into it. You can help them tie a secure knot. Tie a loop on the other end of the string for children to hang on to.

On a mildly breezy day, let children fly their kites on the playground. The short strings allow the kites to fly without getting tangled in power lines or trees.

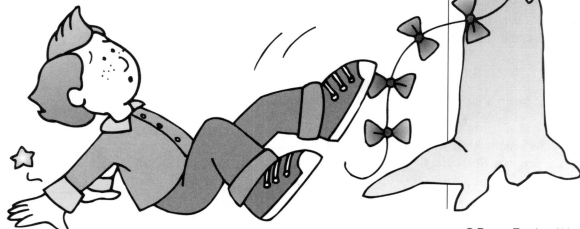

72

Read the following poem to the class. Ask children to write their own kite poems on kite-shaped paper.

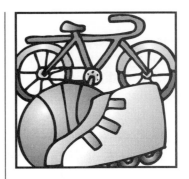

My Kite

I flew my kite up on the hill.
It went straight up as good kites will.
But then, alas! It came back down.
Bop! It landed on the ground.

PLAY BALL!

The Rules	The Reasons
Batters should always wear a batting helmet.	Getting hit in the head with a ball could cause a serious injury.
Catchers should always wear a face mask.	Getting hit in the face with a ball could cause a serious injury.
If a ball goes into the street, let it go. Don't chase it.	It's better that the other team gets a run than that you get hit by a car. Stop! Look! Listen! Remember all safety rules for crossing streets. When it's safe, go get the ball.
When you're at bat, drop the bat after you hit the ball. Do not throw it.	The bat might hit the catcher or another player.
Wait your turn to bat.	Stay far enough away from the batter so you won't get hit by the bat or the ball.

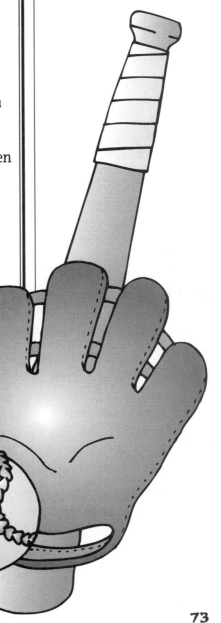

Introduction

Most children are at least vaguely familiar with baseball from seeing it on television or hearing it on the radio. Even very young children enjoy playing bat and ball games, although they may not understand all the rules of baseball. Pitching, batting, and catching are coordination skills that require much practice.

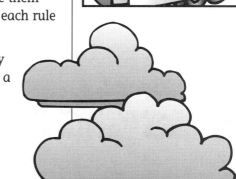

Discussion

Make copies of the "Play Ball!" rules and reasons on page 73 for children. Have them follow along as you read each rule and reason. Ask them to draw a picture for each rule showing the safe way to play.

What is your favorite baseball team? Do you like to play baseball? Why or why not? What position do you like to play? What do you think is a good name for a baseball team?

A TRUE STORY...

Ellie and her friends liked to play baseball. One day Ellie was in the outfield. No one had hit a ball in her direction for a long time. She was bored. Instead of watching the batter, Ellie decided to watch the clouds. Suddenly she heard shouting. Ooops! The ball hit Ellie in the mouth! It really hurt. She had a cut lip and two loose teeth.

What did Ellie do wrong? What should Ellie have done to avoid the injury?

When you're out in the field, watch the game, not the sky or the people in the stands. Is this a good baseball safety rule? Why? What could happen if someone forgets this rule?

Activities

Let children play baseball at recess. The game usually goes quicker if children use a tee or have an adult slow-pitch. Be sure the batter wears a helmet and the catcher wears a face mask.

Divide children into teams for various activities, like spelling bees, math drills or vocabulary quizzes. Ask each team to spend a few minutes deciding on a team name. Have teams write their team name and the names of the team players on a sheet of paper. Each time the teams score a point for a right answer, have them record one run. Teach children to tally runs by drawing four straight vertical lines, then a horizontal line through the four to show five.

Teach children the words to the following song. You may wish to write the words on the board so they can follow along. Sing with children to the tune of "Are You Sleeping?"

I bat safely. I bat safely.
Yes, I do. Yes, I do.
I always wear my helmet. I always wear my helmet.
And you should too. You should too.

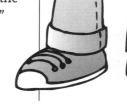

74

Hiking and Camping

The Rules	The Reasons
Always plan your route and stay on marked trails.	Getting lost or spending the night in the woods can be a scary experience when you aren't prepared.
Don't wander off the trail or off by yourself. Stay with your group.	You could get lost. If you fall or get hurt, there won't be anyone to help you.
Be prepared for emergencies.	Even on short hikes, take a small first-aid kit, canteen of water, and a compass.
Plan ahead.	On long hikes, take a map, flashlight, compass, whistle, first-aid kit, food, and water. Dress correctly and take the right equipment.
Streams, rivers, and lakes may look clear and inviting, but don't drink the water.	The water may contain germs that will make you very sick.
Watch the weather.	If an unexpected storm comes up, seek shelter. For more information on thunderstorms and other weather hazards, see Part 6: Outdoor Safety.
Never eat strange plants.	Many types of plants, nuts, berries, and mushrooms are poisonous. For more information on poisonous plants, see Part 6: Outdoor Safety.
Never try to pet, feed, or capture wild animals or birds.	Most wild animals will bite or scratch if you get too close. Mother animals are very protective of their babies. For more information on animal safety, see Part 6: Outdoor Safety.
Leave bees, hornets, and wasps alone. If someone gets stung, put ice on it.	Stings from bees, hornets, and wasps hurt. Whenever possible, stay away from stinging insects.

The Rules	The Reasons

Build only small fires.

Use stones for the base of a campfire.

Make only small fires.

Start fires only in designated areas.

Make sure campfires are completely out before leaving the area.

Never play with matches or lighters.

Review the information on safe fire-building, fire prevention, and putting out fires safely in Part 3: Fire Safety.

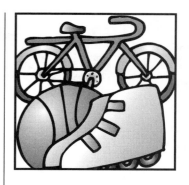

Introduction

Family camping and hiking trips are great ways for children and their parents to share an outdoor experience. The experience will be a pleasant one if everyone follows the safety rules.

Discussion

Have you ever gone hiking or camping? Where did you go? What was it like? What was the best part about hiking or camping? What was the worst part? What could happen if a campfire got out of control?

Activities

Teach or review the four primary directions—north, south, east, and west. Explain what N, S, E, and W stand for on a compass. For older children, add northeast, northwest, southeast, and southwest. Explain the abbreviations *NW, SW, SE,* and *NE.*

Use this opportunity to teach children to use a compass. Bring in several small compasses. Using the compasses, have children find north, south, east, and west. Put up signs on your classroom walls to indicate the four directions.

Ask children to stand, facing north. Then ask children to take turns naming other directions. As each child names a direction, ask the class to turn and face that direction.

Draw this symbol on the chalkboard. Explain how this symbol is like a compass and is used on most maps, to show directions. Provide samples of different types of maps and ask children to find the direction key symbol.

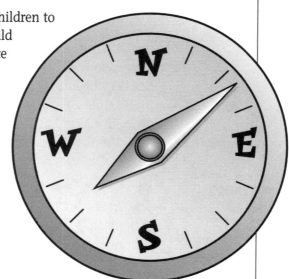

Discussion

Why would it be useful to know which way is south or west? In what direction does the sun rise? In what direction does the sun set?

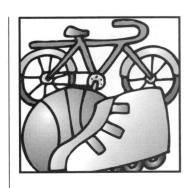

Activities

Ask children to draw pictures of themselves and their families hiking or camping.

Take children on a short nature hike. Ask parents to dress their children appropriately for the field trip. Be sure to review the safe hiking rules before you go, and don't forget to take along a first-aid kit, canteen, and compass.

Invite children to gather acorns, pinecones, hickory nuts, fallen leaves, and other treasures on the hike. Remind them to pick up only items which have fallen to the ground, and not to pick or destroy any plants or flowers.

When children return to the classroom, provide reference books for them to identify leaves, nuts, acorns, and collected treasures. They can glue these items to four-inch white cardboard squares, and label each one to make a nature display in your classroom.

If you can't take children on a field trip, ask them to look for these items in their yards or on their way to school.

You can take children on a "hike" through imaginary woods. Encourage them to use their imaginations and describe what they see along the way. Look up and point to an imaginary bird in a tree. "Look! I see a blue jay! What do you see?" If children look closely, they might imagine rabbits, frogs, snakes, insects, and other small animals along the trail. Have them point out imaginary plants, and beware of the imaginary poison ivy! Don't forget to take a short jump to cross the creek.

After your hike, have the class sit around an imaginary campfire with red, yellow, and orange paper flames, and sing their favorite campfire songs. Let them share a bag of marshmallows or other treat.

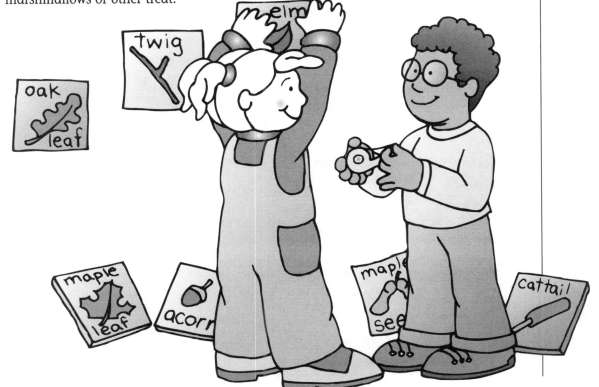

PLAYGROUND SAFETY

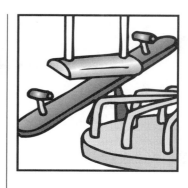

The Rules	The Reasons
Always go to the playground with a friend. Never go alone.	Being with a friend is safer than going alone.

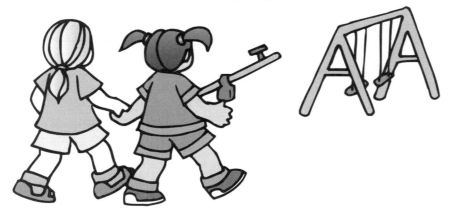

Always let an adult know where you will be.	Never wander off alone. An adult should always know where to find you.
Know where the nearest telephone is located.	In case of an accident, you may need to call for help.
If a storm comes up, go home.	For more information about thunderstorm safety, see Part 6: Outdoor Safety.
Watch out for sharp objects on the playground, like broken glass, nails, or stones.	If you fall, sharp objects could cause bad cuts.
Put your trash in the garbage can.	Keep the playground clear of trash so it is safe for you and your friends.
If a ball rolls into the street, don't chase it. Let it go. Stop, look, and listen before you go into the street.	A driver may not see you if you dash out into the street.

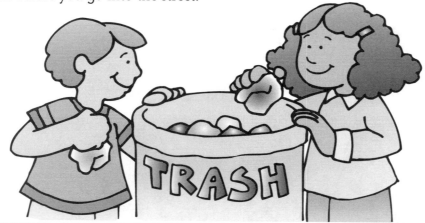

The Rules	**The Reasons**

Hang on tightly when the merry-go-round is moving.

Never jump off the merry-go-round until it comes to a complete stop.

A fall from a fast-moving merry-go-round could cause an injury.

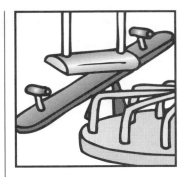

Find an area clear of other people when you jump rope.

You won't accidentally hit anyone with the swinging rope.

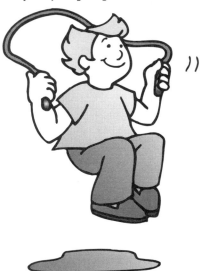

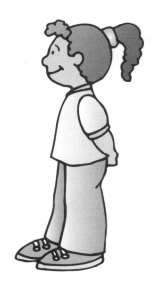

Walk far enough around the swings when other children are swinging.

Then you won't get hit by the children using the swings.

If you see someone getting too close to you when you are swinging, call out a warning.

If you hit someone while you are swinging, the person may be hurt.

Hang on tightly when swinging.

Falls hurt.

Only one person at a time should use a swing.

Two to a swing could cause an accident.

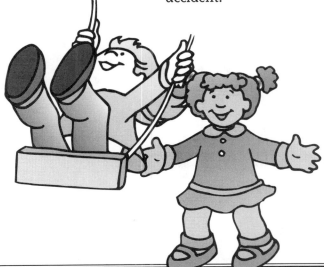

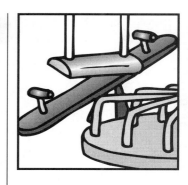

The Rules	The Reasons
Wait until the person in front of you is all the way to the top and sits down before you climb the ladder on the slide.	This will prevent getting accidentally kicked in the face by the person in front of you.
Hold the railing on both sides of the ladder when climbing up the slide.	Falls hurt.
Always go down the slide feet first. Sit on the slide. Don't go down on your stomach or your back.	If you don't sit facing forward, you may not be able to see where you are going.
Never walk up the slide.	Someone coming down could slide into you.

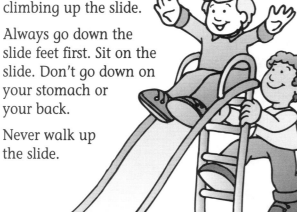

The Rules	The Reasons
Don't get off a teeter-totter suddenly when the other person is up in the air.	The other person may fall. The teeter-totter may come up suddenly and hit you in the chin.
Hang on tightly to the handle with both hands.	
Sit frontwards, not backwards.	You may fall off.
Don't stand on the teeter-totter.	
Don't throw sand or dirt.	It may get in someone's eyes.

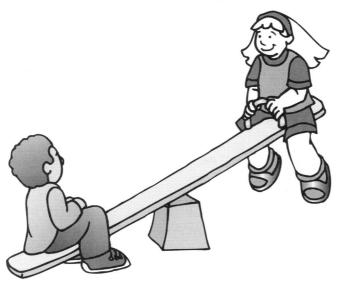

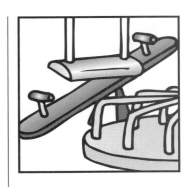

Introduction

Playing at a playground is fun, but getting hurt isn't. Safety rules on the playground help you and your friends play safely.

Discussion

Copy and distribute the "Playground Safety Rules and Reasons" on pages 78–80. Go through each rule and reason as children follow along. Point to the illustrations for each safety rule. Ask children to give their own reasons or examples for why these are good rules. Ask them if they can think of any other safety tips to add to this list.

Why are safety rules important on the playground? Have you ever seen an accident on a playground? What happened? How did it happen? How could it have been prevented?

Activities

Invite children to color the "Playground Safety Rules and Reasons" pages and take them home to share with their families.

Make a copy of the activity sheet, "Safety at the Playground" on page 82 for each child. Let children complete the activity individually. Then go through it with the class, asking children to share which items they circled and why. If children missed some items, encourage them to circle the correct answers at that time.

Have children make playground safety posters. Display them in the hall outside your classroom or near the doors leading to the playground.

While children are playing on the playground at school, this is a good opportunity to "catch them doing something right." Safety Award certificates (see page vi) can be issued to children who follow the safety rules.

Swings, slides, teeter-totters, merry-go-rounds, and climbing equipment are commonly found on many playgrounds and in neighborhood parks. Ask children to brainstorm ideas for other types of non-mechanical equipment which might be fun to have at a playground. Divide the class into small groups. Have each group draw an illustration of a new type of playground equipment, based on their ideas.

Ask children to name words that rhyme with "play" (anyway, bay, birthday, bray, Broadway, cay, caraway, day, display, gay, gray, hay, hurray, Jay, Kay, lay, May, may, nay, pay, pray, ray, say, someday, stay, tray, way, Monday, Tuesday, Wednesday, etc.) Write the words on the board as they name them. Using words from the list, or other words that rhyme with "play," ask children to write a two-line rhyming poem. Children can title and illustrate their poems.

Example:

When I went out to play with Kay
I saw a brightly colored blue jay.

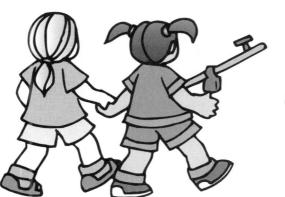

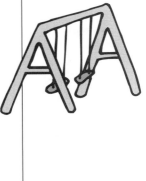

Safety at the Playground

Study the picture below. Circle all the parts of the picture that show children following playground safety rules.

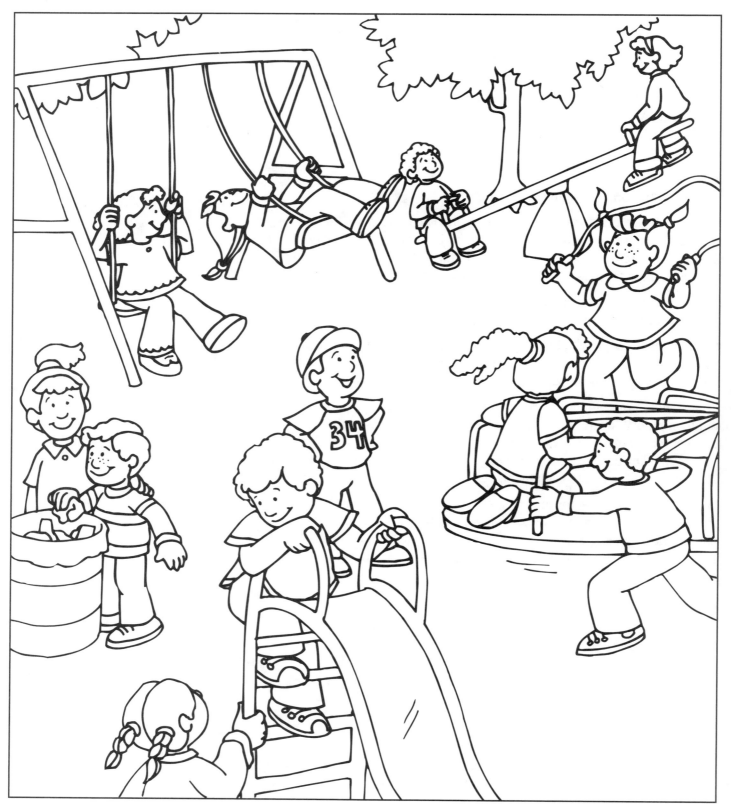

Reproducible © Fearon Teacher Aids FE7959

WATER SAFETY:
SWIMMING, DIVING, AND WATERSKIING

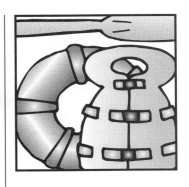

The Rules	The Reasons
Learn to swim.	By learning to swim, you will be safer in the water. Take lessons from an instructor, and practice with adult supervision.
Always swim where there is a lifeguard or responsible adult to supervise.	If you get in trouble, it's best to have someone close by to help.

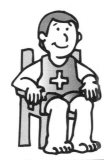

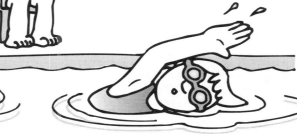

The Rules	The Reasons
Don't distract lifeguards by talking to them while they are on duty.	The lifeguard's job is to stay alert and watch for swimmers in trouble.
Swim only in areas where swimming is permitted.	Don't swim in quarries, ditches, or other unsafe places. The water may contain sharp objects or dangerous chemicals.
If a storm comes up or you can see lightning, even if it's far away, get out of the water. If you're in a boat, head for shore immediately.	Water conducts electricity from lightning.
Don't try to rescue someone yourself.	Leave rescues to those who are trained. You can help by throwing a life preserver or other floating object. Yell for help immediately.

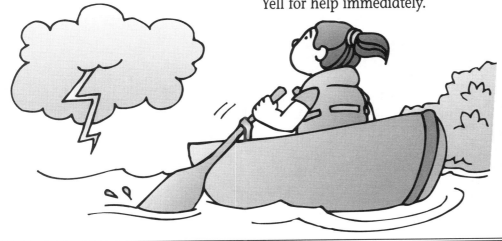

The Rules	The Reasons
Don't swim near docks or in areas where there are boaters or water skiers.	A boater or person on water skis might not see you in the water.
Be aware of sharp objects in the sand.	Shells, stones, or trash can cut your feet. It's a good idea to wear shoes or sandals on the beach.
Pick up your trash to keep the beach safe for yourself and others.	

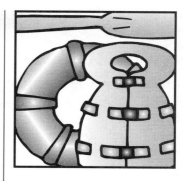

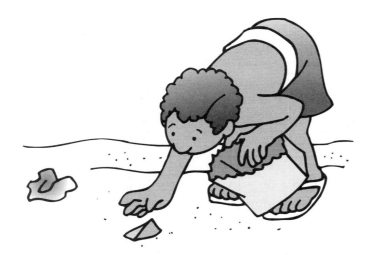

Always wear life jackets at the beach.	A large wave could knock you over or push you under the water.
Never throw sand.	It might get in someone's eyes.
At pools, hold on to the railing when you go in and out of the pool.	Wet steps are slippery.

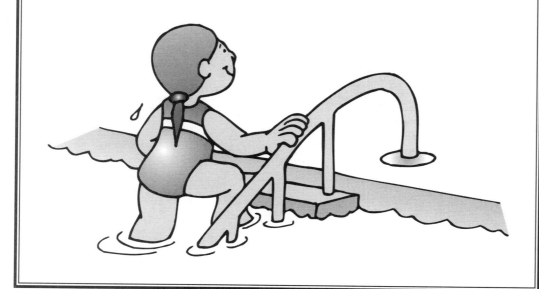

The Rules	**The Reasons**

Never run along the outside of the pool or in the locker area.

Wet floors are slippery too.

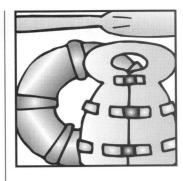

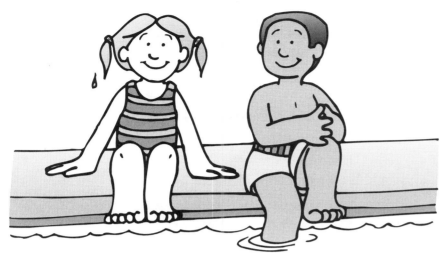

Don't play or swim in the area under the diving board.

Someone on the diving board may not see you below and could land on you. You both could get hurt.

Never jump into a pool from the sides.

You could land on someone and hurt him or her or hit your head on the side of the pool.

Never push anyone into a pool or into the water from a raft, boat, or dock.

The person may not know how to swim. The person could bump his or her head on the raft, boat, or dock.

Obey all the signs at the beach or pool where you swim.

The signs are for your protection.

Always swim with another person nearby.

When you swim with a buddy, you can watch out for each other and call for help if the other person gets in trouble.

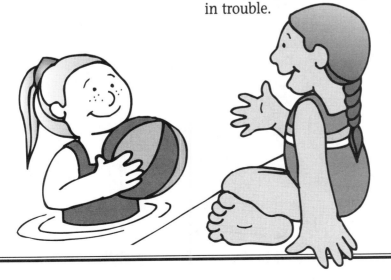

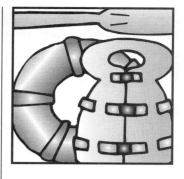

The Rules	The Reasons
Don't swim after eating a large meal. Wait at least 30 minutes before going into the water.	Swimming too soon after eating could cause stomach cramps.
Stay out of water deeper than your head when swimming.	Even if you know how to swim, deep water can be dangerous. Wait until you become an experienced swimmer.
Learn to swim before you try to learn to dive.	You need to be in water over your head when diving.
Dive only in deep water.	If you dive in shallow water you could hit the bottom and get hurt.
Dive only with an experienced lifeguard or adult diver present.	Diving can be dangerous. Learn to do it the right way so you don't get hurt.

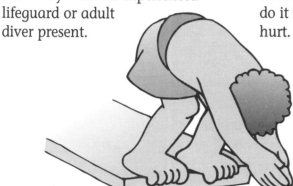

Dive only in areas set up for diving. Do not dive off docks or tree branches.	The water may not be deep enough. There may be stones, trees branches, or other obstacles in the water.
Always wear a life jacket when you water-ski.	If you fall, the life jacket will keep you afloat.
Learn to swim before you try to water-ski.	You need to be in water over your head when water-skiing.
Ski behind a boat driven by a responsible adult.	Driving a boat while someone is water-skiing can be difficult. For your safety, the driver should be experienced.

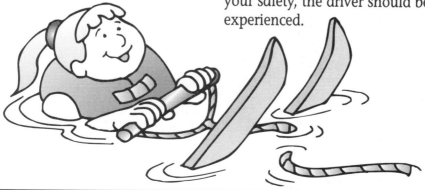

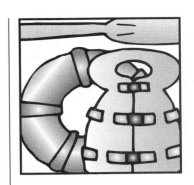

Introduction

Swimming, diving, wading, fishing, boating, and water-skiing are great ways to have fun in the water. If you learn the safety rules for playing in or near the water, you can have fun and be safe, too. Remind children to use the buddy system when swimming.

Discussion

Do you know how to swim? How did you learn? Where do you like to swim? What is the buddy system? Why is it important not to go into the water alone?

Activities

A field trip to an indoor pool would be a great way to reinforce the safety rules children have learned.

Invite a lifeguard or certified swimming instructor to speak to the class about water safety. Encourage children to ask questions and participate in the discussion.

Have a "day at the beach" in your classroom or on the playground. Play beach games, like volleyball, with a beach ball. Invite children to build sand castles. Top off the day with hot dogs, chips, and sodas.

To reinforce the water-safety rules, ask children to fill in the blanks with *NEVER* or *ALWAYS* as you read each sentence. This can be done by asking individuals or groups.

_____ swim with a friend.

_____ swim with a lifeguard or responsible adult present.

_____ swim alone.

_____ push someone in the water from the side of a pool.

_____ hold on to the railing when going in or out of a pool.

_____ swim in areas marked *NO SWIMMING*.

_____ wear a life jacket while in a boat.

_____ swim under the diving board.

_____ dive in water that is deep enough.

_____ pick up your trash on the beach.

_____ dive off of docks, rafts, or boats.

_____ throw sand.

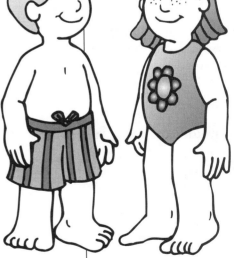

If a storm comes up while you are swimming, you should _____ get out of the water.

_____ run along the outside of a pool or locker room.

WATER SAFETY: BOATING AND FISHING

The Rules	The Reasons
Always wear a life jacket.	If the boat overturns or you fall overboard, the life jacket will keep you afloat.
Don't overload a boat or raft.	It might sink.
Don't lean over the side of a boat or raft.	You might fall out.
Only a responsible adult should drive a motorboat.	For everyone's safety, children should never drive a motorboat.
No horseplay in a boat.	Someone may fall overboard.
When riding in a motorboat, be sure there is a fire extinguisher onboard. Learn how to use it.	A spark from the engine may start a fire.
Never go barefoot in a boat.	Wet decks are slippery.
If a boat turns over in the water, stay with the boat until help comes.	It will be easier for a rescuer to spot you in the water if you are near the boat. You can hang onto the boat to help stay afloat.
If a storm comes up or you see lightning while you are out in a boat, go to shore immediately.	A storm can cause large waves which may cause the boat to capsize. Water conducts electricity from lightning.
Always wear a life jacket when you fish from a boat or pier.	A life jacket will keep you afloat if you fall in the water.
Follow all boat-safety rules when fishing from a boat.	Safety rules will keep you safe.
Be careful when handling fishhooks.	Fishhooks are sharp. If you get a fishhook in your hand, let an adult remove it.
If your fishing line gets snagged, let an adult help get the line free.	Tugging on a snagged line could cause you to lose your balance. You could fall.

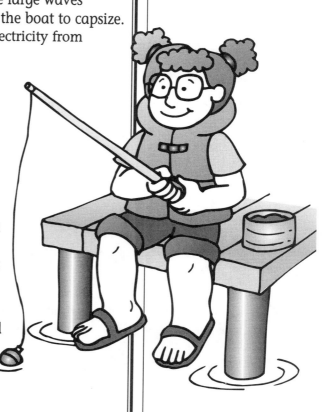

Discussion

Have you ever gone fishing or boating? Where did you go? What kind of fish did you catch? Did you wear a life jacket?

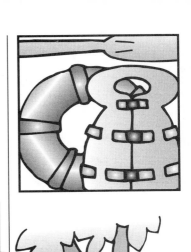

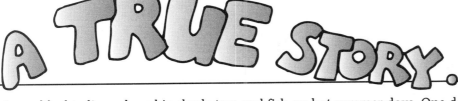

Jason liked to lie under a big shade tree and fish on hot summer days. One day he cast his line and his lure got caught in the tree branches above him. He tugged and tugged, but couldn't get it free. He decided to climb the tree. When he got part way up, a duck nesting in the tree quacked at him. This startled him and he fell out of the tree. He landed on the rocks below. Not only did he break three fingers on his hand, he never did get the lure out of the tree.

What did Jason do wrong? What could Jason have done differently?

Activities

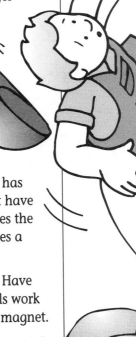

Invite children to make a water safety bulletin-board display. Make copies of pages 90–92. Use the enlarger feature on the copier if you have it. Have children cut out the patterns and write a water-safety tip on each one. They can decorate the pictures with crayons, markers, and colored pencils.

On a rainy day when they can't play outside, teach children to play the card game *Go Fish*. With young children, use a half deck of regular cards, two of each card. Divide children into groups of three or four. Deal four cards to each child. Spread out the remaining cards face down in the middle. Have children search their cards for pairs. When children get a pair, have them set the cards aside. Children take turns asking other players for a specific card. For example, Sue could ask, "Alex, do you have any twos?" If Alex has a two, he gives it to Sue. She makes a pair and takes another turn. If Alex doesn't have a two, he says, "Go fish." Sue then takes one card from the "fish" pile. If it matches the number she asked for, she makes a pair and asks again. If not, the next child takes a turn. The first player to match all the cards in his or her hand is the winner.

Children can make their own fishing poles and go fishing right in the classroom! Have them tie a 36-inch piece of string to a 24-inch dowel. (Quarter- or half-inch dowels work well.) At the other end of the string, tie a small magnet or one-inch piece of strip magnet.

Photocopy the patterns on pages 90–92. Make several copies so there will be enough fish for each child to have at least two. Let children cut out the fish and color them with markers or crayons. Tape or glue a one-inch piece of strip magnet to each fish. Put the fish in a pail or cardboard box. Let children "go fish."

For cross-curriculum activities, write a math problem or new reading word on each fish. Let children take turns fishing. When a child catches a fish, ask him or her to answer the math problem or read the word. If the child answers correctly, he or she keeps the fish. If not, the fish must be thrown back.

Fish Patterns

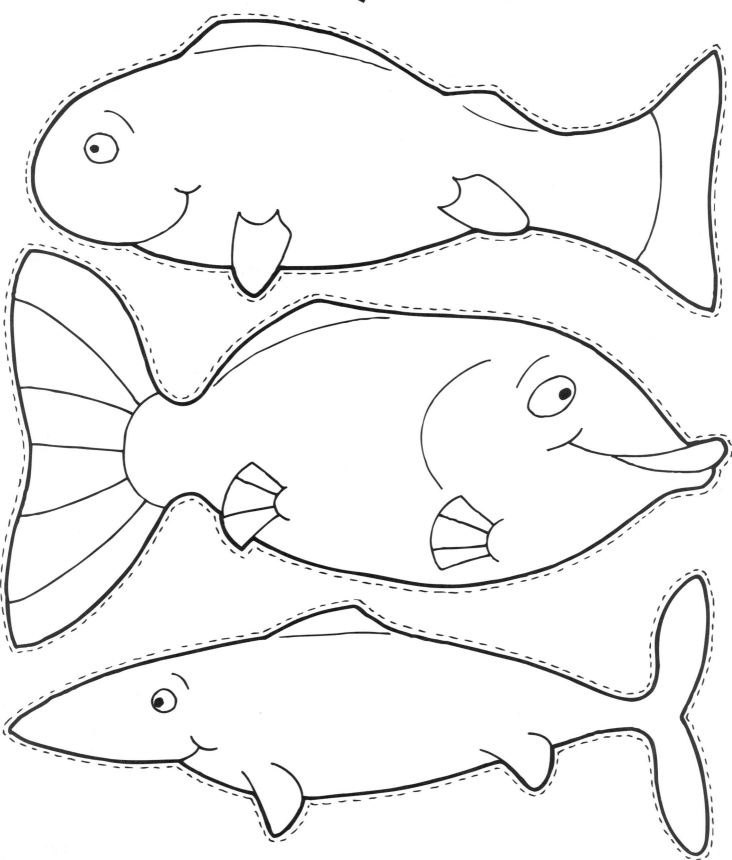

Beach Patterns

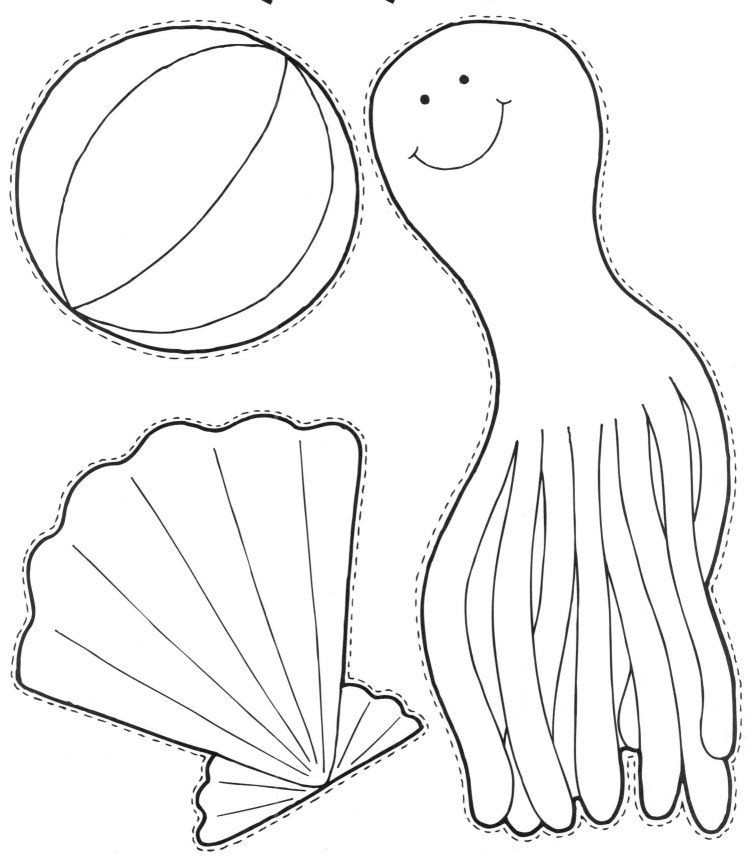

Reproducible

Beach Patterns

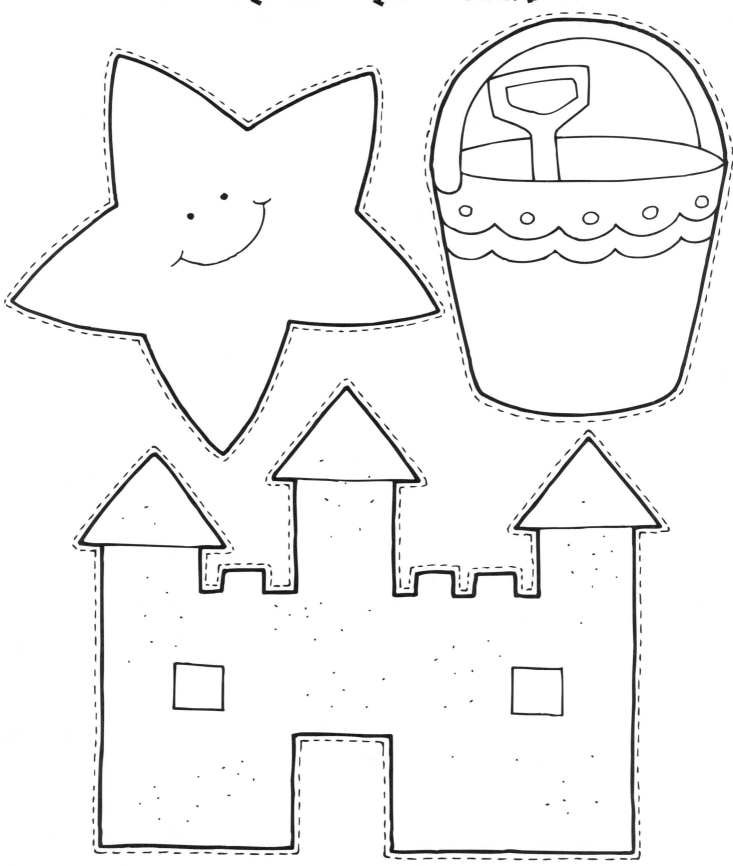

Reproducible

SLEDDING SAFETY

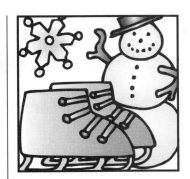

The Rules	The Reasons
Be aware of obstacles when sledding. Don't sled where you might run into trees or rocks.	Sledding is fun. Crashing isn't fun. Running into trees or rocks while going down a hill can cause injuries.
Check what's at the end of the hill when you go sledding, before you get to the bottom.	Is there a road or street at the bottom of the hill? Stop your sled before you end up in the middle of traffic.

ICE-SKATING SAFETY

The Rules	The Reasons
Skate only at skating rinks or at supervised ponds. Never skate on a pond if you see open water.	Thin ice on an unsupervised pond can break. Falling into icy water in winter can be dangerous.
Never walk or skate on thin ice.	You could fall into freezing water. Pay attention to signs which warn of thin ice.
Dress warm enough for the weather.	Skating won't be any fun if you are too cold to enjoy it.

Introduction

One of children's favorite sports in the winter is sledding. As soon as a few inches of snow fall, children head for the nearest hill. Some use fancy sleds, others slide on a piece of cardboard. Sleds can travel very fast down a steep hill.

Safety experts suggest that young children wear helmets when sledding for protection in case they fall or run into a rock or tree.

Discussion

Have you ever gone sledding or ice-skating? Where did you go? What was it like? Why would it be a good idea to wear a helmet when sledding? What other winter activities do you enjoy?

What happens to ice when the weather gets warm? Did you know the sun can cause ice to melt even when the temperature is below freezing? Why is ice dangerous when it is thin? What could happen if you fell through the ice? If there is ice on a pond, how cold do you think the water will be?

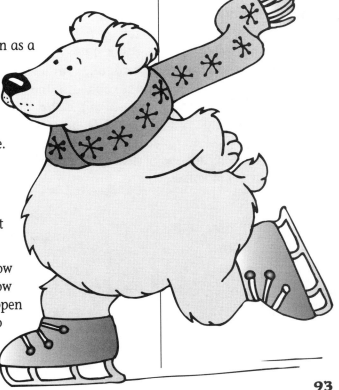

93

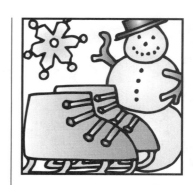

Activities

Let children do experiments with water and ice.

- Have children fill a small plastic bucket and ice-cube tray with water and place them in a freezer. How long does it take for the water to freeze? Which froze first, the water in the bucket or the water in the ice-cube tray? Why?

- Set a tray of ice cubes on a windowsill inside the classroom. If possible, set another tray of ice cubes outside the window on a sunny winter day. Have children observe happens to the ice when the sun shines on it.

- Fill two large plastic glasses or jars half full of water about the same temperature. Take the temperature of the water and record it for both containers. Add ice cubes to one container. Have children take turns taking the temperature of both containers every ten minutes over a several hour period. Have children record their results. Which container is colder? How much colder? How long did it stay colder? How long did it take before the water in both containers was the same temperature again?

Let children cut out pictures from old magazines to make a sports safety collage.

Make a copy of the activity sheet, "Sports Safety Is for Everyone" on page 97 for each child. Invite children to complete the activity individually. Then go through it with the class, asking children to tell which items they added and why. If children missed some items, encourage them to add them at that time.

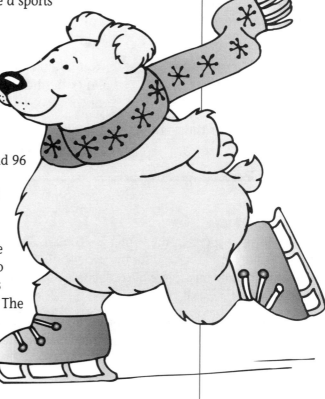

Play Sports Safety Concentration. Photocopy pages 95 and 96 on heavy paper or light cardboard. Make several sets so children can play in small groups. Cut out the cards and mix them up. Place the cards in rows, face down. You may want to use only five or six sets of cards for very young children. The first child turns over two cards. If the cards match, the child keeps the cards and turns over two more. If the cards do not match, the child turns the cards face down again and play continues with the next child. The game ends when all pairs are matched. Shuffle the cards and play again. If you have the resources, make one set of cards for each child in the class to take home and play with their families.

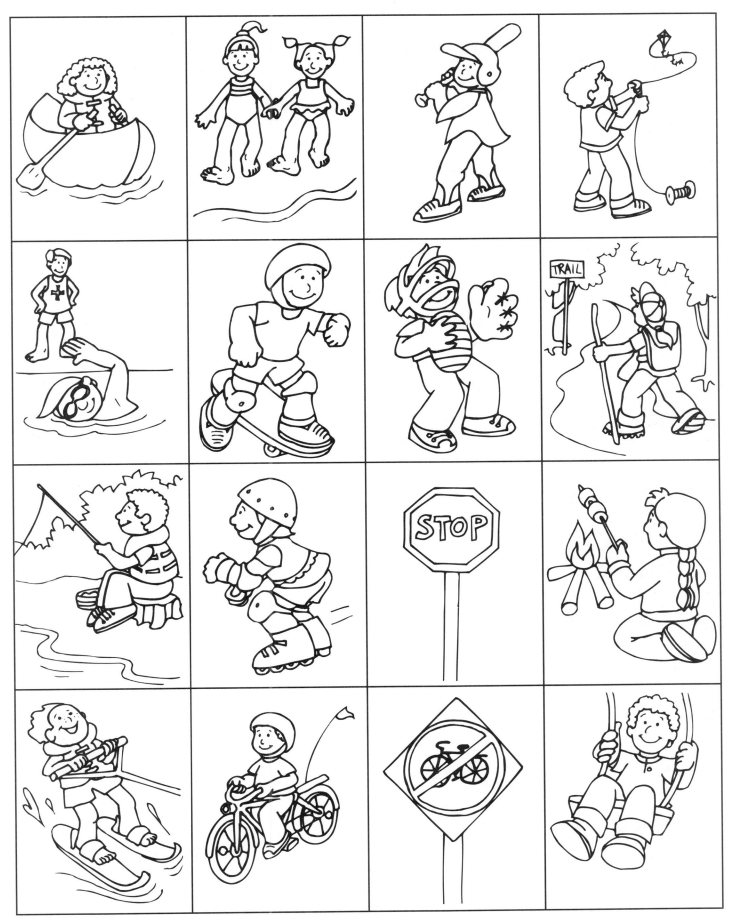

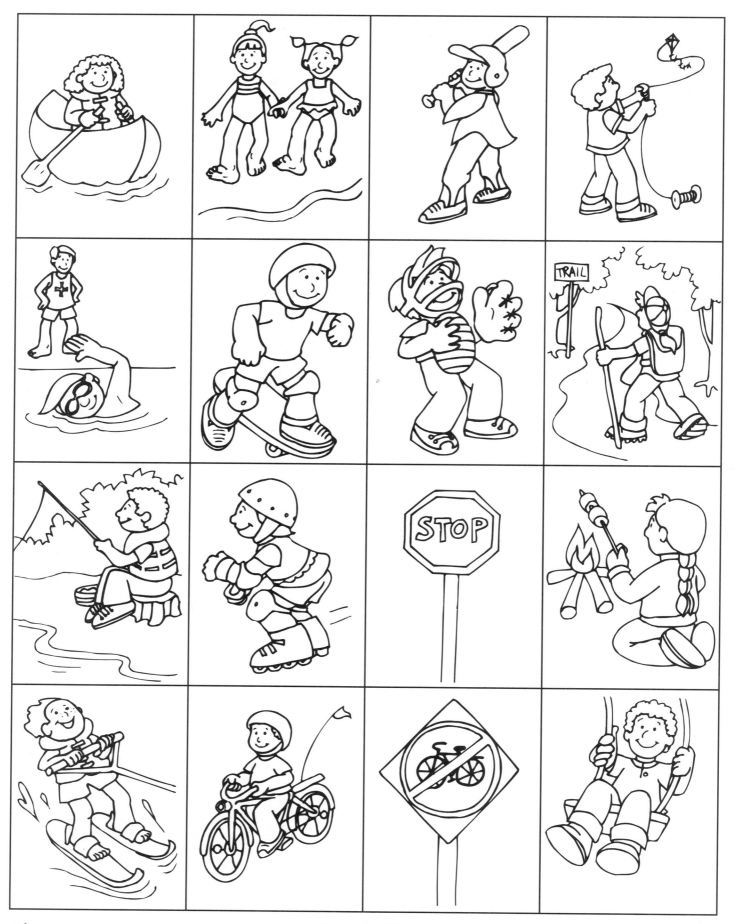

Reproducible

Sports Safety Is for Everyone

What is missing from each picture? Draw in the missing items to help these children play safely.

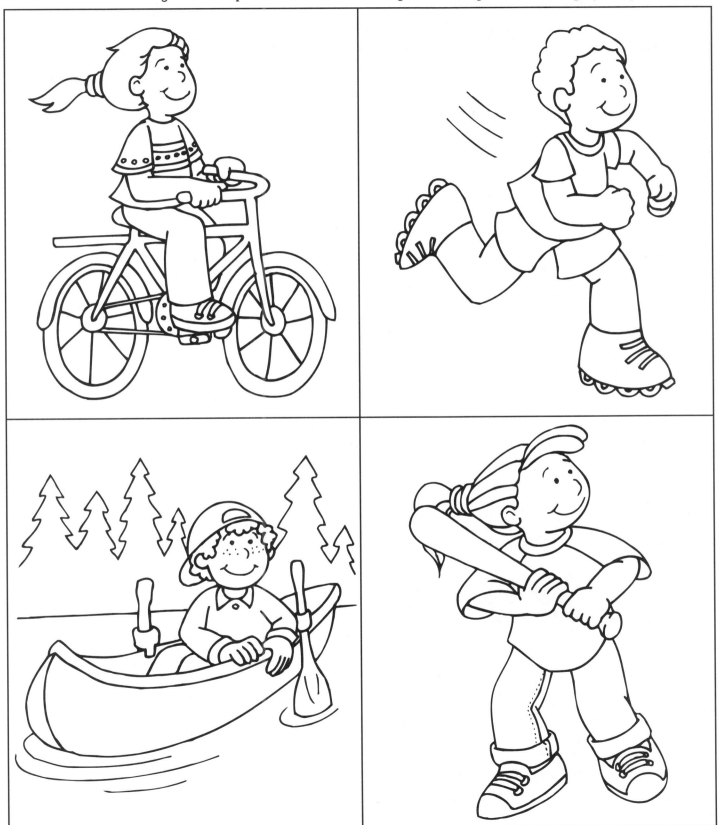

OUTDOOR SAFETY

CROSSING STREETS SAFELY

The Rules	The Reasons
Never run into the street. Cross only at the corner or at marked crosswalks.	A car may not be able to stop in time if the driver doesn't see you coming.

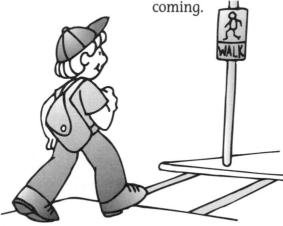

The Rules	The Reasons
Stop at the curb. Look left. Look right. Look left again.	By looking both ways, you will know if a car is coming from either direction.
Watch for turning cars, buses, motorcycles, and trucks. Listen for cars coming that you might not be able to see.	If you hear a car coming fast, wait for it, even if you can't see it. Someone driving fast will not be able to stop quickly.
Listen for sirens. Never try to cross the street when an emergency vehicle is coming with sirens on, even if the walk sign is lit and the light is green.	When fire trucks, ambulances, and police cars have their sirens on, that means they are in a hurry. They always have the right of way.

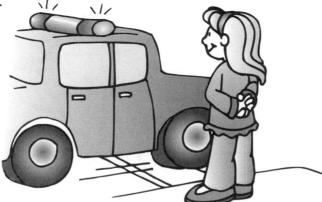

The Rules	The Reasons
Don't dawdle. Cross quickly, but don't run.	You might slip or trip and fall if you run.

The Rules	The Reasons

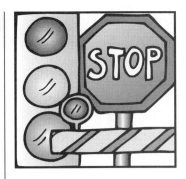

When it is icy or wet, be extra careful crossing streets.

Rain and snow can make sidewalks and roads slippery. When it rains or snows, drivers have a harder time seeing you. They also have a harder time stopping quickly. Wait until cars come to a complete stop.

At traffic lights, wait for the green light or WALK signal.

The green light or WALK signal means it is safe to cross.

Stop at driveways. Watch for cars backing out.

Drivers may not be able to see you when they back out of driveways.

Always obey crossing guards.

Crossing guards help us cross busy streets safely.

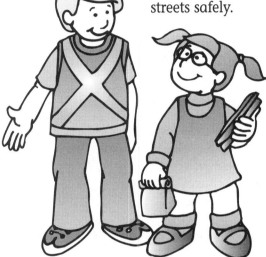

Never play in or near streets.

Streets are not good places to play because of traffic.

If there are no sidewalks, always walk on the left side of the road, facing traffic. Stay as far off the road as possible.

Drivers will be able to see you better if you are facing them as you walk.

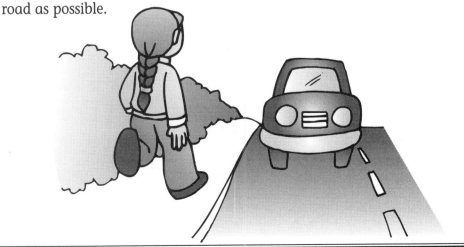

Introduction

Children cross streets every day going back and forth to school, stores, and playgrounds. They need to be extra careful crossing busy streets. If a child gets hit by a car, bus, truck, or motorcycle, he or she could be badly hurt. Knowing the rules for crossing streets safely and following them will keep you safe.

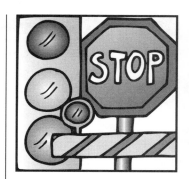

Discussion

Make copies of the "Crossing Streets Safely Rules and Reasons" on the two previous pages 98 and 99 for children. Read through the rules and reasons as they follow along. Encourage children to discuss the rules and reasons. Ask them to give examples or situations that relate to each rule.

If the stoplight is green, but you see a car coming fast, what should you do? Which side is the left side of the street?

Activities

Have children practice learning left from right.

Take a walk with your class as a group. Review the safety rules for crossing streets safely as you go.

Set up a pretend street on a tabletop. Let children use toy cars and small people figures to act out the rules for crossing streets safely.

Ask children to make up short slogans about crossing streets safely. Help them write their slogans neatly on large square, rectangular, or triangular pieces of yellow construction paper. They can decorate them with black markers to look like street signs. Display the safety signs in your classroom or in the hall outside your classroom.

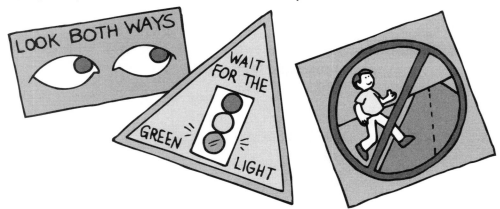

Teach children the words to the following song. You may wish to write the words on the board so children can follow along. Sing with children to the tune of "Are You Sleeping?"

> *I cross streets safely.*
> *I cross streets safely.*
> *Yes, I do.*
> *Yes, I do.*
> *I stop, and look, and listen.*
> *I stop, and look, and listen.*
> *And you should too.*
> *You should too.*

108

RIDING THE BUS

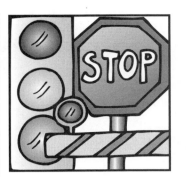

The Rules	The Reasons
Don't distract the driver.	The driver must watch for traffic signs, cars, trucks, motorcycles, bicycle riders and people walking.
Keep the noise level low.	The bus driver must listen for sirens and other traffic sounds.
Wait until the bus comes to a complete stop before getting off or on.	You could fall if the bus is moving.
Hold on to the handrail. Stay seated while the bus is moving.	Holding the handrail and staying seated while the bus is moving also helps prevent falls.
Don't run out in front of the bus while it's stopped.	Wait for the bus to leave so you have a clear view of traffic.

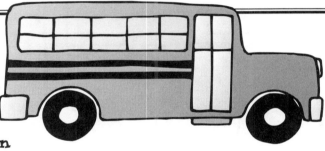

Introduction

The bus driver is responsible for the safety of all the people riding the bus. Obeying safe bus-riding rules helps the driver do his or her job.

Discussion

Do you ever ride a bus? Where do you go on a bus? Have you ever taken a long bus ride to another city? Are the rules for riding a school bus the same as the ones for riding the city bus? How is a bus like a car? How is it different?

Activities

Invite a school bus driver to speak to your class. Encourage children to ask questions and participate in the discussion.

Take the class on an imaginary bus ride. Arrange chairs four across with an "aisle" down the middle. Let children take turns being the bus driver. Others can take turns getting off and on the bus, remembering to hold the imaginary handrail and walk behind the bus before crossing the street.

Make copies of the bus pattern on page 102. Use yellow paper if available. Have children cut out the bus and write a bus-safety slogan on the side of the bus. They can decorate the bus with crayons or markers. Encourage them to add children riding in the bus. Display the busses in your classroom.

School-Bus Pattern

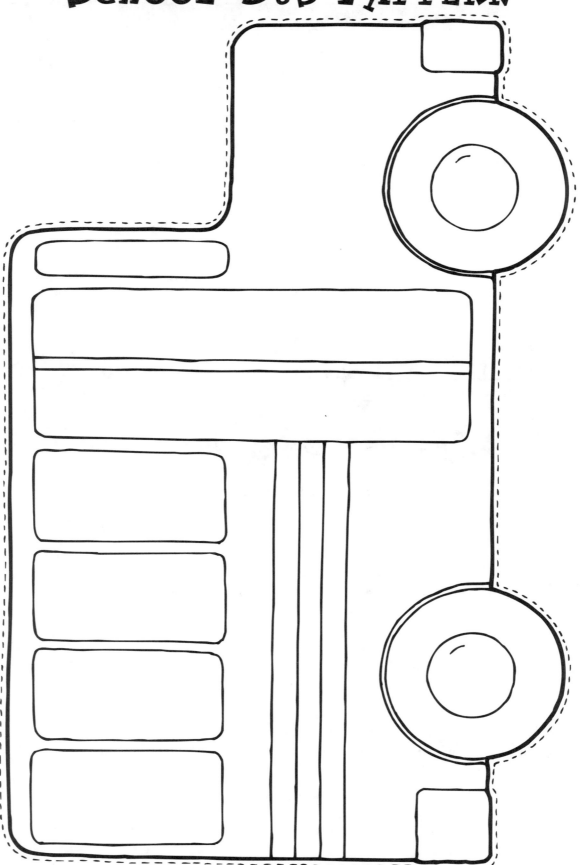

Reproducible

RIDING IN A CAR

The Rules	The Reasons
Always wear your seat belt.	Seat belts protect passengers in case the driver stops quickly or the car is in an accident.
In cars with air bags on the passenger side of the front seat, always sit in the back seat.	The force of the air bag may injure you in an accident. Children under 12 should sit in the back seat.
Babies and very young children need to sit in a special car seat.	Car seats keep children safer if an accident happens.
Don't distract the driver.	The driver must watch for other cars, people walking, and traffic signs. You can help by talking or playing quietly and not bothering the driver.
Keep your head, hands, and feet inside the car at all times.	If another vehicle passes too close to your car, or if your car gets too close to a wall or fence, you could be injured.

Introduction

Cars are great for going long distances or for getting to nearby places quickly. The driver of a car must obey many safety rules. People who ride in cars need to obey safety rules, too. Knowing these safety tips for riding in a car can make trips safer for you, the driver, other passengers, and other cars on the road.

Discussion

What are some safety rules drivers must obey? How can you help the driver? How can you help younger children be safe while riding in the car? If someone gets in your car and doesn't put the seat belt on, what should you do? What safety rules would you need to know if you are riding in a taxi? How are the safety rules for riding in a bus and a car alike? How are they different?

Activities

Here is another rule for safe riding in a car: *When leaving the car, check for traffic before opening the door. On busy streets, get out of the car on the curb side.* Ask children to give the reason for this rule.

Invite children to make their own "bumper stickers." Give each child a sheet of colored paper about four inches wide and 12 to 18 inches long. Ask children to make up a safe driving slogan and write it on the bumper sticker. Display the bumper stickers in your classroom. Let children vote on the best bumper-sticker idea.

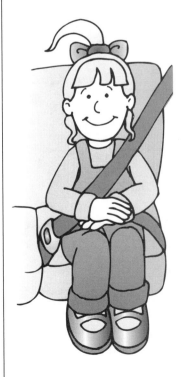

SAFETY CHARADES

Make a copy of pages 104 and 105. Cut out the slogans. Fold them in half and place them in a box. Let children take turns picking a slogan and acting it out without using any words, while classmates guess the slogan. Add your own slogans or safety tips. Whisper the slogan to children who haven't learned to read yet.

STOP! DROP! ROLL!

STOP! LOOK! LISTEN!

BUCKLE UP FOR SAFETY!

ONLY YOU CAN PREVENT FOREST FIRES

ALWAYS WEAR A BIKE HELMET

KEEP BOTH HANDS ON THE HANDLEBARS

DON'T EAT STRANGE PLANTS

STAY AWAY FROM STRANGE ANIMALS

DON'T WALK OR RIDE WITH STRANGERS

THINK BEFORE YOU ACT

ALWAYS SWIM WITH A FRIEND

NEVER PLAY WITH MATCHES

FIRECRACKERS ARE NOT TOYS

ALWAYS WEAR A LIFEJACKET IN A BOAT

KEEP POISONS LOCKED AWAY

PRACTICE FAMILY FIRE DRILLS

KEEP STAIRS CLEAR OF TOYS

WIPE UP SPILLS

Reproducible

Safety Charades

WEAR A HELMET WHEN YOU BAT

CROSS ONLY AT CORNERS

STAY SEATED ON THE BUS

KEEP YOUR BIKE IN GOOD REPAIR

KNOW YOUR FAMILY CODE WORD

DRESS WARMLY WHEN IT IS COLD

USE SUNSCREEN WHEN IT IS HOT

GO INSIDE DURING A THUNDER STORM

STAY OUT OF WATER WHEN IT IS LIGHTNING

CROSS THE STREET WHEN THE LIGHT IS GREEN

FLY KITES AWAY FROM POWER LINES

NEVER RUN INTO THE STREET

WATCH FOR TURNING CARS

WATCH FOR CARS BACKING OUT OF DRIVEWAYS

OBEY CROSSING GUARDS

DON'T DISTRACT BUS DRIVERS

STAY SEATED ON THE BUS

DON'T PLAY ON RAILROAD TRACKS

RAILROAD TRACKS MEAN TRAINS

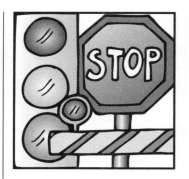

The Rules	The Reasons
Don't play on or around railroad tracks.	It takes a long time for a train to stop.
Watch for railroad signals when riding your bicycle.	Most tracks have flashing lights and gates that lower before the train comes through. Usually trains blow their whistles before approaching an intersection.
Stop, look, and listen before you cross the tracks.	A train may be coming even though you can't see it. You should be able to hear it if you stop and listen.
If you see or hear a train coming, never try to beat the train across the tracks.	The train might be coming faster than you think.

Introduction

Riding on a train or subway is a great adventure, but remember—trains travel at high speeds. They cannot stop quickly. Playing around railroad tracks is not a safe idea.

Discussion

Have you ever been on a train? What was it like? Where did you go? Do you like riding trains? If you have never ridden on a train, what do you think it would be like? Why do you think it takes much longer for a train to stop than it does for a car or truck?

Activity

Help children "get aboard the safety train." Make a copy of the train engine on page 107. Cut it out and display it on a bulletin board or tape it to the wall. Make copies of the train-car patterns on pages 107 and 108, one car per child. Ask children to cut out the train cars and write a traffic-safety slogan—anything related to crossing streets safely, riding in a car or bus safely, or being safe around railroad tracks. Have them decorate the cars and sign their names. Add the cars to the display behind the engine.

Invite children to "become" trains. One child can be the engine. The others can "follow the leader" around the gym or playground, copying the actions and sounds of the leader. Let children take turns being the leader and the caboose.

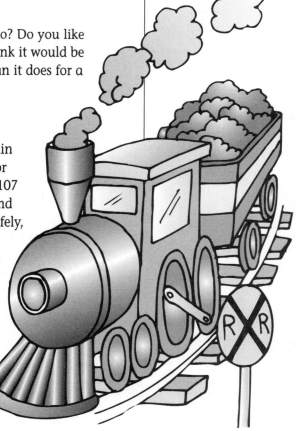

106

Train Pattern

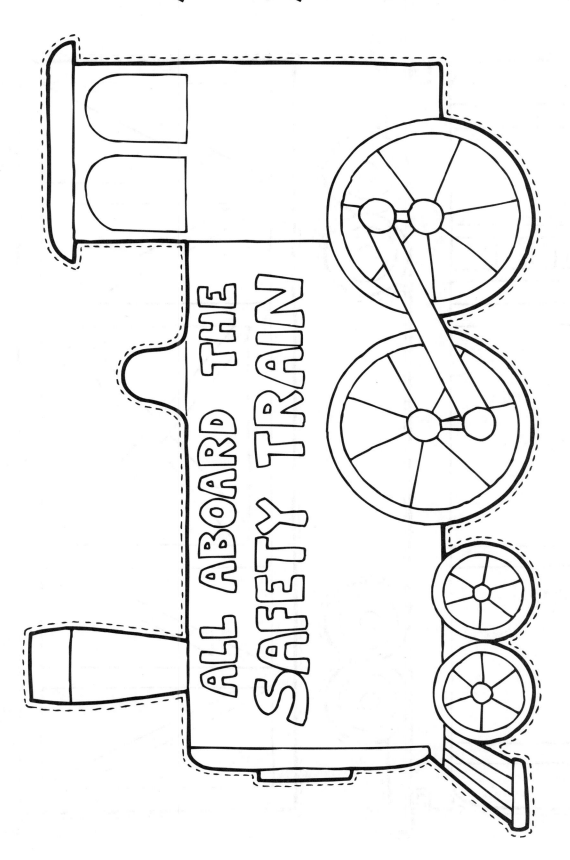

ALL ABOARD THE SAFETY TRAIN

Reproducible

Train Patterns

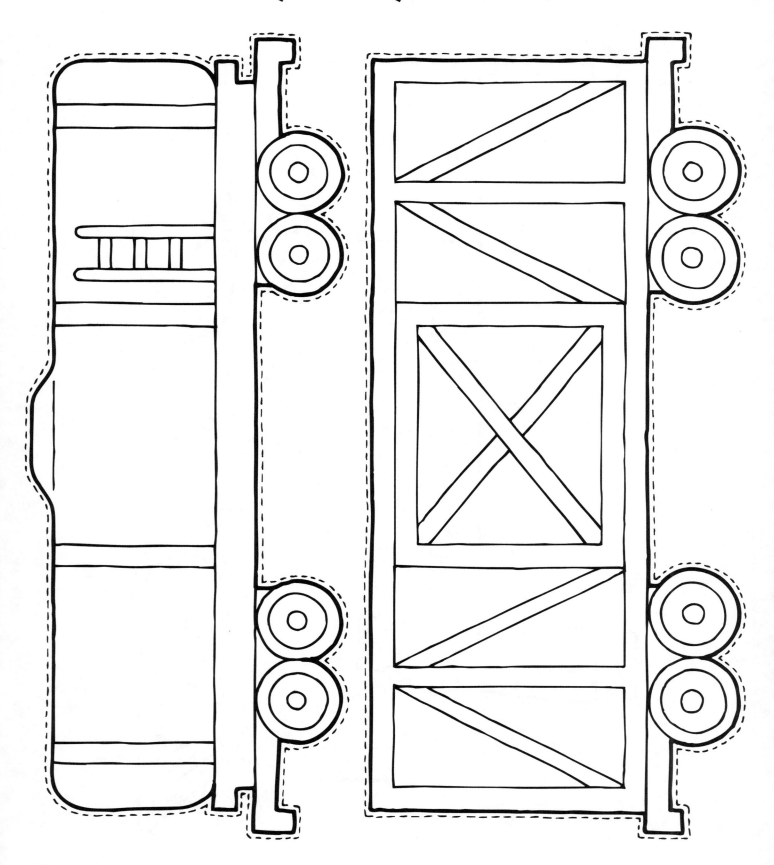

Reproducible

Plants, Trees, Mushrooms, Nuts, and Berries

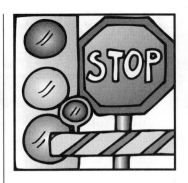

The Rules	The Reasons
Do not eat any plants, nuts, mushrooms, or berries unless you know for sure they are safe.	Many types of plants are poisonous.
Do not pick unfamiliar plants, flowers, or mushrooms.	Some plants cause skin rashes, itching, and burning. Some have sharp spikes or thorns.
Do not climb tall trees or climb on thin branches.	If you fall, you could be injured or cut badly.

Introduction

Wild berries and fruits, flowers, and plants can be pretty to look at, but many are poisonous. Stay away from unfamiliar plants. Some are poisonous, like poison ivy and poison oak. They can cause rashes, itching, and burning. Some plants have thorns or spikes that can poke you. Many types of plants, berries, nuts, and mushrooms are poisonous.

Discussion

If you find a bush with some bright, juicy-looking berries on it, what should you do? If the birds are eating the berries, does that mean it is safe for you to eat them, too? (NO!)

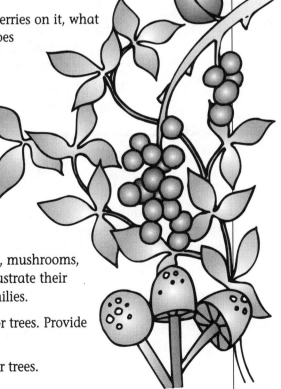

Activities

Read the following poem to the class.

Please Don't Eat the Flowers

Look at the lovely flowers.
Sniff them if you please.
But don't eat the berries,
Mushrooms, flowers, or trees.

Ask children to make up short poems about flowers, mushrooms, berries, fruit, vegetables, nuts, or trees. They can illustrate their poems and take them home to share with their families.

Use this opportunity to introduce a unit on plants or trees. Provide reference books for identification.

Ask children to draw their favorite types of plants or trees.

ANIMAL SAFETY

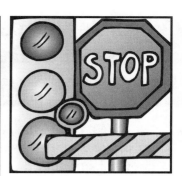

The Rules	The Reasons
Be very careful around a mother animal and her babies.	The mother may think you are trying to hurt her babies. Even animals that are tame can be dangerous if they think their babies are in danger.
Never pet a strange animal, play with it, or feed it.	Some animals are not friendly. If the animal isn't your pet, stay away from it.
Stay away from an injured animal, even if it is your own pet.	When an animal is hurt, it may be scared and may not recognize you. It could snap or bite. Call an adult to help.
When animals are eating, leave them alone.	Even pets may bite if they think you are trying to take their food away.
Wild animals are fun to watch, but leave them alone.	Even a squirrel or a rabbit can bite if you try to catch it.
Don't tease any animal.	You might get bit.
Don't feed strange animals.	You might get bit.
Stay away from stinging insects.	Stings from bees, hornets, and wasps hurt. Ask an adult to check and see if the stinger is still in. If you get stung, put ice on it right away.

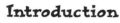

Introduction

Children often want to pet "cuddly"-looking animals, or make friends with dogs and cats they meet. Some animals are not friendly. Most wild animals will not allow you to touch them, and all can bite or scratch, even the friendliest-looking ones.

Discussion

Many accidents are caused by unsafe actions and could have been prevented. If a driver is going too fast around a corner and runs into a tree, that is called an accident. But if the driver had been going slower, the accident could have been prevented.

116

Read each of the following scenarios to the class. Ask children to describe the unsafe action and how the accident could have been prevented. Ask children to make up or relate some real-life accidents that were caused by unsafe actions and could have been prevented.

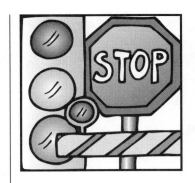

- When Joe finished raking, he left the rake in the yard. His dad didn't see it. He tripped and fell.

- Jan saw a cute puppy wandering around in her back yard. She went up to it and tried to pet it. The puppy bit her.

- Carlos forgot to wear his seat belt. When his mother had to stop suddenly, he hit his head on the dashboard.

- Rachel didn't wear her bike helmet. As she was riding, she hit a bump in the road and fell off her bike. She ended up with a big bump on her head.

- Terry found a bee hive. "I wonder if there is any honey in there?" he thought. He started poking at the hive. That caused hundred of angry bees to come out of the hive. Terry was stung four times before he could run away from the bees.

If you get stung by a bee and don't have any ice, what else could you use? (Apply a cold can of soda, a package of frozen peas, or a Popsicle™.)

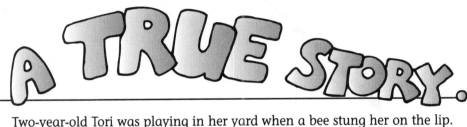

Two-year-old Tori was playing in her yard when a bee stung her on the lip. Her mother wiped away her tears and gave her a Popsicle™ right away. Then she checked to make sure the stinger was out.

Why was it a smart idea for her mother to give Tori a Popsicle?™ (Ice reduces swelling from a sting.)

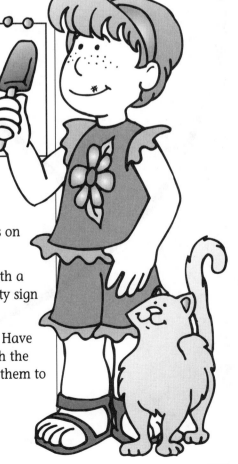

Activities

Have children cut out pictures from old magazines that show people following outdoor safety rules. Children can work in groups to make outdoor safety collages on large pieces of posterboard.

Make a copy of the "No" sign on page 112 for each child. Explain that a circle with a line through it means "NOT to do something." Ask each child to make a NO safety sign relating to some aspect of outdoor safety.

Make a copy of the "Unsafe Actions Cause Accidents" activity sheet on page 113. Have children complete the activity independently. When they finish, go through it with the class. Ask children to show the safe action they drew for various pictures and ask them to explain why that action is safe.

"No" Sign

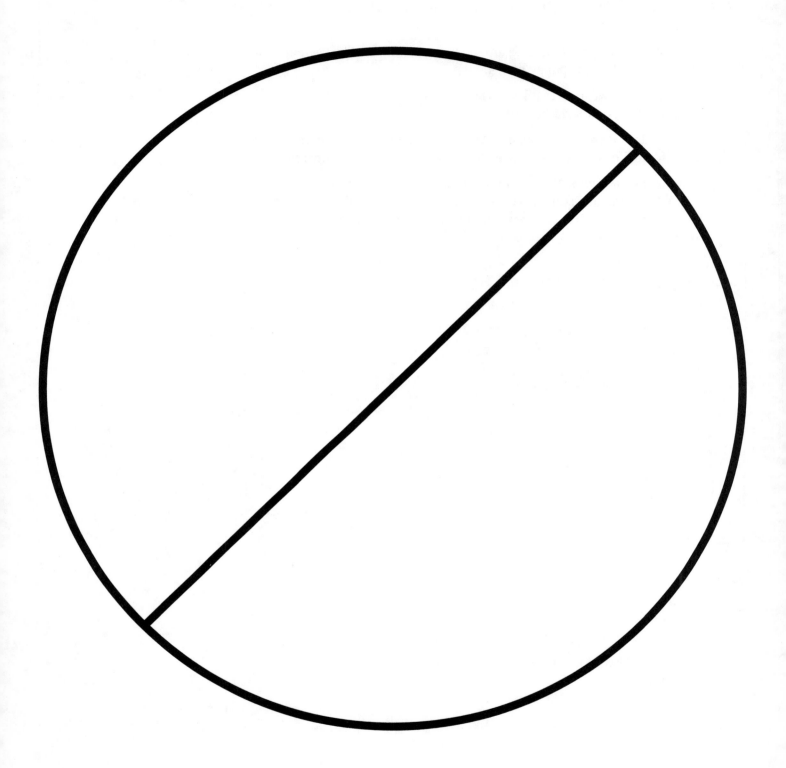

UNSAFE ACTIONS CAUSE ACCIDENTS

Look at the pictures of unsafe actions. For each unsafe action, draw a picture to show a safe action.

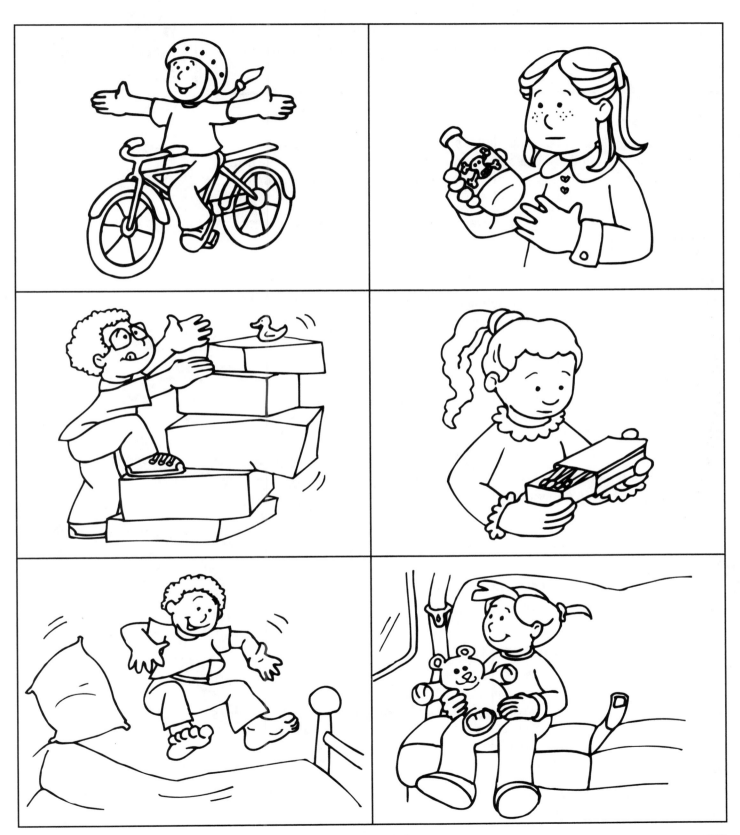

Beat the Heat

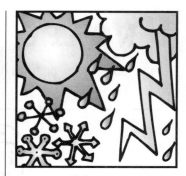

The Rules	The Reasons
Protect yourself from sunburn. Use sunscreen. Wear a hat. If your skin turns pink, get out of the sun.	Sunburn can be very painful. When your skin begins to turn pink or feel hot to the touch, you may be in danger of burning.

Introduction

Playing outside in the summer is fun, but if you're outside too long when it's hot, you could get a sunburn. Sunburn can occur even when it is cloudy. When you are near water, the sun reflects off the water and you can burn more quickly. After swimming, reapply sunscreen if needed.

When you sweat, your body loses moisture. Drink plenty of liquids, especially water, on hot days. Getting too hot can also cause heatstroke and you could become very sick.

Discussion

What activities do you enjoy on hot summer days? Did you ever get sunburned? How did it feel? What do you do to keep cool in hot weather? If you have pets, what should you do to keep them safe from the heat?

Activities

Read the labels on several types of sunscreen to the class. Explain the meaning of SPF (sun protection factor). An SPF of 15 means it will give 15 times more protection than bare skin and is the minimum recommended.

Bring an outdoor thermometer to class. Use this opportunity to demonstrate how to read a thermometer.

Ask children to draw pictures of themselves doing something they enjoy on a hot summer day.

Ask children to make a list of words that rhyme with "hot" (*cot, dot, got, jot, lot, not, knot, pot, spot, rot, tot, shot, slot, plot, blot, clot, trot, forgot, jackpot, robot,* and *Scott*).

Read the following poem to the class:

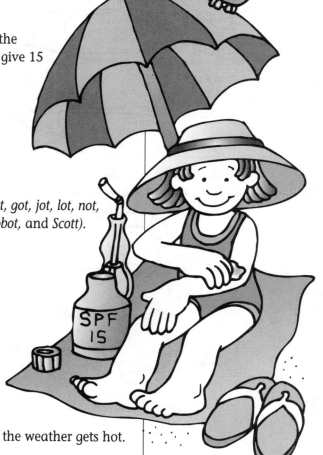

When It Gets Too Hot

When it gets too hot
I find a spot
That's nice and shady and cool.
I get out of the sun
And have some fun
Reading by the pool.

Have children write their own short poems about what to do when the weather gets hot. Ask children to illustrate their poems.

114

BRRRRR ... BEWARE OF THE COLD

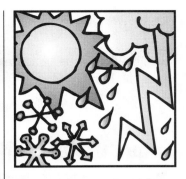

The Rules	The Reasons
Dress warmly during cold weather. Go inside when you begin to feel cold.	Frostbite can be very dangerous and painful.
Dress in layers.	This will keep you warmer. If you get too warm, you can always take off some layers.
Stay inside during a bad snowstorm or blizzard.	Whiteouts can occur during a blizzard. A whiteout means the blowing snow makes it difficult to see even a few feet ahead. You could easily get lost, even close to your home.

Introduction

Sledding, skiing, ice-skating, and building snow people are great winter activities. Hats, boots, mittens, scarves, and hoods can protect you from the cold and prevent frostbite. Being dressed warmly is more important than being fashionable.

Frostbite can occur in a short time during very cold weather.

Even the warmest jackets can let cold air in. Dressing in layers keeps warm air in and cold air out. Boots should be waterproof or water resistant to keep feet dry.

Be prepared for a big snowstorm or blizzard by watching weather reports.

Discussion

What winter activities do you enjoy? Does it snow where you live? What activities can children enjoy when it snows? What do you do to keep warm when it is very cold? If you have pets, what should you do to keep them safe from the cold?

Activities

Provide a variety of boy and girl dolls and clothing or paper dolls and clothing. Let children dress the dolls appropriately for different types of weather.

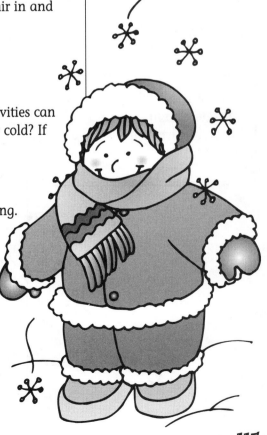

Invite the school nurse or other appropriate medical personnel to speak to your class about sunburn, heatstroke, hypothermia, and frostbite. (Choose whichever topic is appropriate, depending on where you live and the time of year.) Encourage children to ask questions and participate in the discussion.

Invite a veterinarian, someone from the local humane society, or a pet-store employee to speak to your class about pet safety in hot and/or cold weather. Encourage children to ask questions and participate in the discussion.

Ask children to make a list of words that rhyme with "cold" *(old, bold, told, mold, old, blindfold, hold, behold, Harold, billfold, gold, sold, marigold,* and *unfold).*

Have children write sentences using as many words as they can that rhyme with "cold." Example: *Harold told me he folded a marigold in his old billfold.*

After a fresh snowfall, let children go outside and make snow angels.

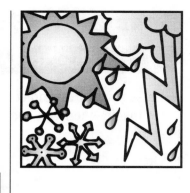

Lightning Is Beautiful . . . and Dangerous

The Rules	The Reasons
Stay away from water during a thunderstorm. If you are swimming, get out of the water. Do not take a bath or shower during a thunderstorm.	Lightning is attracted to water. It is not a safe place to be in a thunderstorm.
If you are outside, go inside. If you can't go inside, stay away from metal objects, like fences, pipes, and poles.	Objects like fences, pipes, and poles can carry electricity from lightning.
Don't stand under a tree that is alone in a field.	Lightning usually strikes the highest object in an area. If you're in a big field, crouch down. Don't be the highest object.
If you're in a car, stay there.	A car is safe in a thunderstorm.
Stay away from windows.	Lightning can strike through glass.
Use the telephone during a thunderstorm only in an emergency.	The telephone can conduct electricity from lightning.
Do not use a television with an outside antenna during a thunderstorm.	The television antenna can conduct electricity from lightning. Listen to weather reports on the radio.

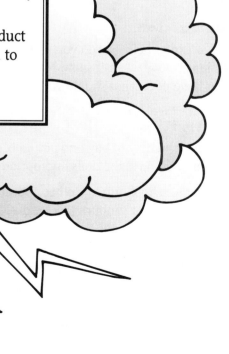

116

Introduction

CRASH! BAM! RUMBLE! BOOM! Thunder is loud and scary, but it can't hurt you. Lightning may be beautiful, but it can be dangerous. Lightning can start fires in houses, barns, or forests. It may knock over trees or power lines.

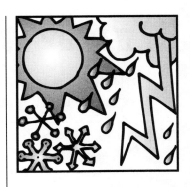

Storms come up quickly sometimes. Watch the sky. If the wind comes up suddenly or the clouds begin to get very dark, a storm may be coming. Go inside. Listen to weather reports.

Discussion

How do you feel when there is a thunderstorm? Why should you stay away from windows during a storm? If the power goes out during a storm, what should you do? Why would it be better to use a flashlight than a candle for light if the power goes out?

Too much rain can cause floods. Does that mean rain is bad? Why do we need rain? What would happen if it never rained?

Activities

Use this opportunity to introduce a unit a weather.

Invite a meteorologist to speak to your class about how thunderstorms are formed and what causes thunder and lightning.

Encourage children to ask questions and participate in the discussion.

Let children make their own thunderstorm. Darken the room. Divide children into three groups. One group can use flashlights to imitate lightning. Another group can make a variety of sound effects to imitate thunder by using a large wooden spoon to hit the inside of a cardboard box, beating on a drum, or crashing cymbals. Let children think of other ways to imitate the sound of thunder. The third group can imitate the sound of wind and the rain.

Make a copy of the "Whatever the Weather—Be Prepared"activity sheet on page 118 for each child.

Ask children to make thunderstorm safety posters.

Ask children to make up sentences using words that rhyme with "rain." For example, *The rain in Spain falls mainly on the plain.*

Ask children to draw pictures showing how rain helps plants, animals, and people.

Play Weather Safety Concentration. Photocopy pages 119 and 120 on heavy paper or light cardboard. Make several sets so children can play in small groups. Cut out the cards and mix them up. Place the cards in rows, face down. You may want to use only five or six sets of cards for very young children.

The first child turns over two cards. If the cards match, the child keeps the cards and turns over two more. If the cards do not match, the child turns the cards face down, again, and play continues with the next child. The game ends when all pairs are matched. Shuffle the cards and play again.

If you have the resources, make one set of cards for each child in the class to take home and play with their families.

Whatever the Weather—Be Prepared

Help these children dress for the kind of weather shown in each picture. Draw a line from the children to the clothing they should wear to be safe.

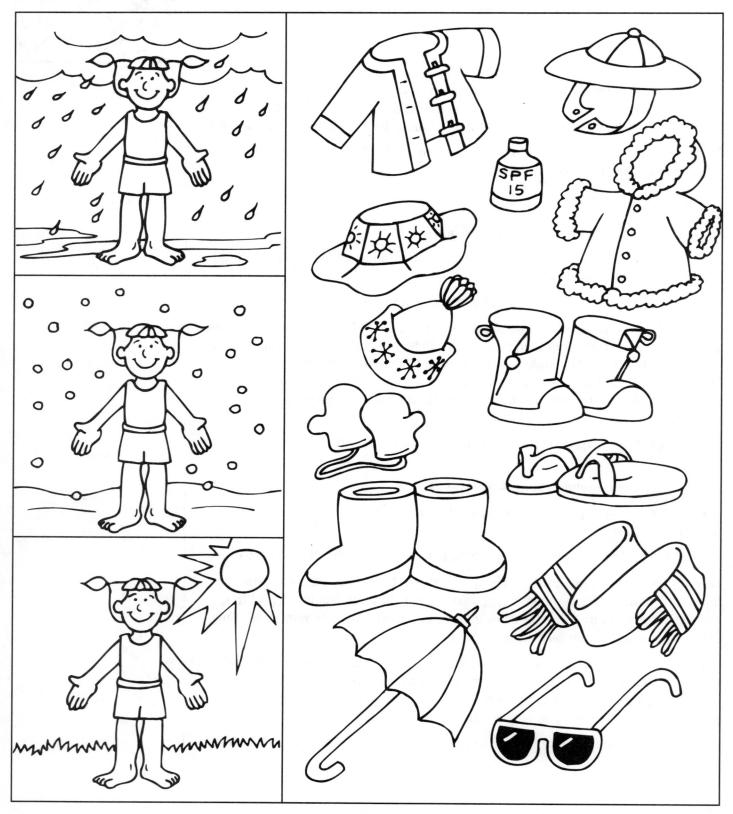

Reproducible

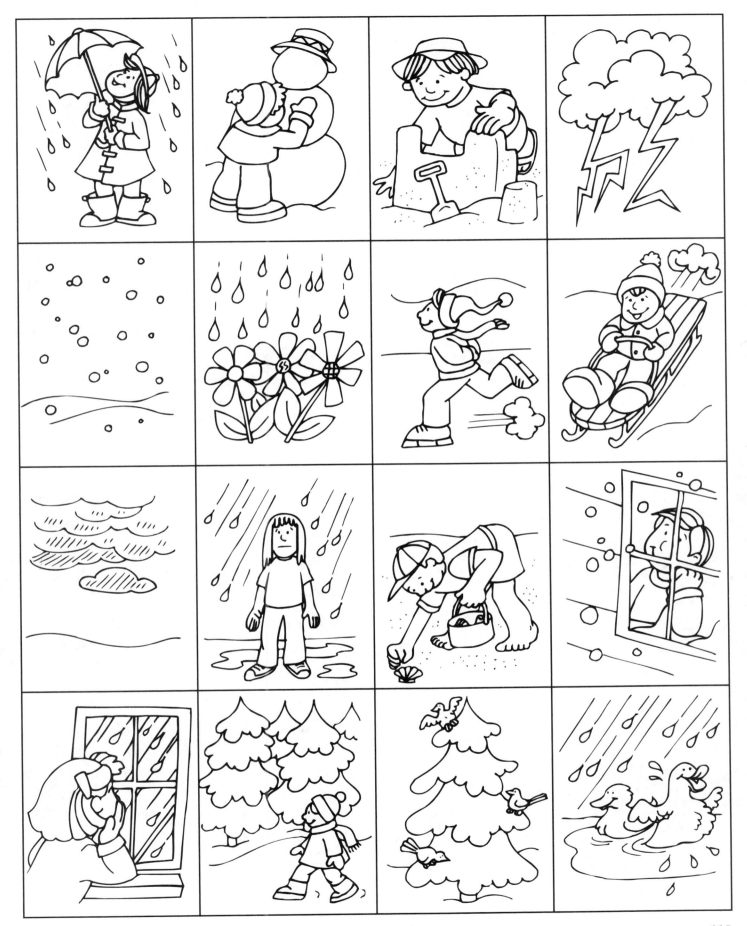

Reproducible

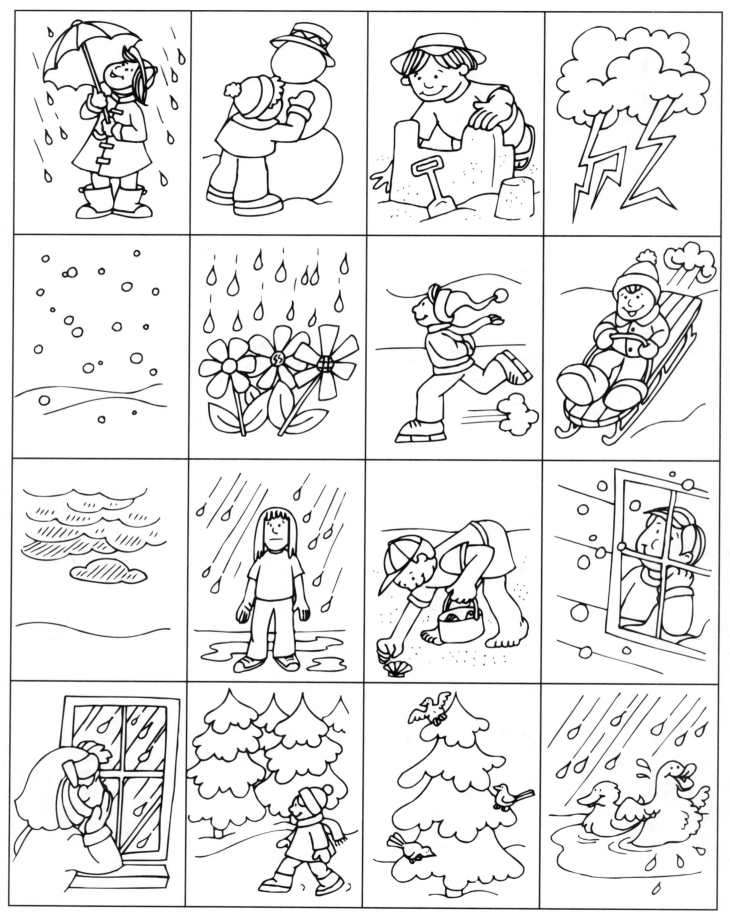

© Fearon Teacher Aids FE7959

Terrible Tornadoes

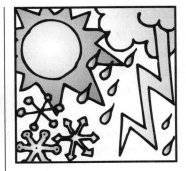

Note: If tornadoes do not occur in the area where you live, you may wish to skip this section with your class.

The Rules	The Reasons
Learn the meaning for a tornado watch and a tornado warning.	A **watch** means conditions are right for a tornado. A watch usually lasts for an hour or more.
Go to a safe place immediately when a tornado warning is issued.	A **warning** means someone has seen a tornado or one is showing up on radar. Go to a safe place immediately.
	The best place to go when a tornado warning is issued is a storm cellar or the southwest corner of your basement. Under the stairs or a strong work bench is also a safe place to be. If you do not have a basement, go to an inner room without windows, like a bathroom.
	If you are in a mobile home, get out. Go the the nearest shelter if there is time. If not, lie face down in a ditch. Cover your head with your hands. By going to a ditch or low spot, you may be protected from flying sticks and objects blown by strong winds.
	If you are outdoors, lie flat in a low spot, like a ditch. If you are in a car, leave the car and go to the lowest spot. A car is not safe during a tornado. Lie flat and cover your head.
	If you are at school, follow directions. Go quickly to the proper place, but do not run. Walk quietly so you can hear directions.
	Keep away from windows and metal objects since lightning usually occurs when there is a tornado.
Be prepared.	Keep a battery radio and flashlight in the place where you will go if a tornado occurs. Make sure the batteries are working.
Do not use the telephone unless there is a major emergency.	The telephone can conduct electricity from lightning.

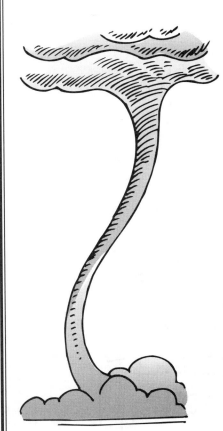

Introduction

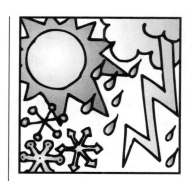

About 1,000 tornadoes occur in the United States each year. Tornadoes are terrible storms that can cause much damage to property. People who are not in a safe place can be injured. Most tornadoes happen during March, April, and May, but they can occur any time of the year.

During a tornado watch, stay tuned to your radio or TV. Check the batteries in your flashlight and portable radio. Know where you should go if the weather gets worse. Bring pets inside for protection.

The intensity of tornadoes and other severe wind storms are measured on the Fujita scale (also called the F scale) created by T. Theodore Fujita. The scale uses numbers from zero to five, based on the amount and type of wind damage.

Category	Wind Speed	Damage	Strength
F-0	Up to 72 MPH	Light	Weak
F-1	73–112 MPH	Moderate	Weak
F-2	113–157 MPH	Considerable	Strong
F-3	158–206 MPH	Severe	Strong
F-4	207–260 MPH	Devastating	Violent
F-5	261+ MPH	Incredible	Violent

Discussion

Many people say that a tornado sounds like a freight train. If you hear a sound like that during a storm, what should you do? (Head for shelter immediately.)

A tornado often looks like a huge funnel cloud coming out of the sky. What should you do if you see a cloud that looks like a huge funnel? (Same answer as above.)

Activities

Hold tornado drills so children know where to go and what to do if a tornado warning is issued while they are at school.

Send home copies of the Parent Letter/Tornado Safety Tips on page 123 for children to share with their families. Encourage children to discuss an emergency plan and practice tornado drills at home with their families.

Many books about tornadoes show excellent pictures of funnel clouds. Gather books or pictures of tornadoes and share them with the class so children know what funnel clouds look like.

If tornadoes occur frequently in your area, invite someone from the local emergency government or appropriate organization to speak about what to do during a tornado watch and warning. Encourage children to ask questions and participate in the discussion.

Dear Parents,

Tornadoes are terrible storms that can cause much damage to property and injure people who are not in a safe place. Most tornadoes happen during March, April, and May, but they can occur any time of the year.

We have discussed tornado safety in class. Please review the tornado safety tips below with your family. Nothing can be done to stop a tornado, but being warned and following the tornado safety precautions can prevent injuries and save lives.

Tornado Safety Tips

When there is danger of a tornado, a watch or warning will be announced on the TV and radio. A **watch** means conditions are right for a tornado. A watch usually lasts an hour or more.

During a watch, stay tuned to your radio or TV. Check the batteries in your flashlight and portable radio. Know where you should go if the weather gets worse. Bring pets inside for protection.

A **warning** means someone has seen a tornado or one is showing on radar. Go to a safe place immediately.

Many people say that a tornado sounds like the roar of a freight train. If you hear a sound like that during a storm, head for shelter immediately.

The best place to go if a tornado warning is issued is a storm cellar or the southwest corner of your basement. Under the stairs or a strong work bench is also a safe place to be. If you do not have a basement, go to an inner room without windows, like a bathroom.

If you are in a mobile home, get out. Go to the nearest shelter if there is time. If not, lie face down in a ditch. Cover your head with your hands. By going to a ditch or low spot, you may be protected from flying sticks and objects blown by strong tornado winds.

If you are outdoors, lie flat in a low spot, like a ditch. Never try to outrun a tornado in a car. If you are in a car, leave the car and go to the lowest spot. A car is not safe during a tornado. Lie flat and cover your head.

Keep away from windows and metal objects since lightning usually occurs when there is a tornado. Do not use the telephone except in an extreme emergency.

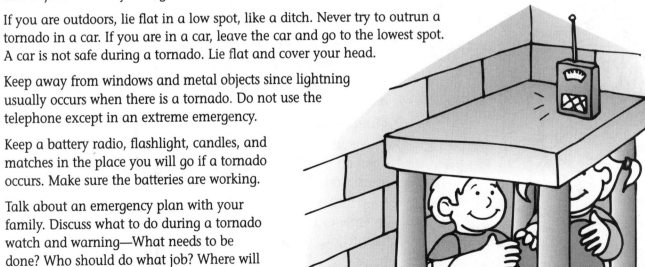

Keep a battery radio, flashlight, candles, and matches in the place you will go if a tornado occurs. Make sure the batteries are working.

Talk about an emergency plan with your family. Discuss what to do during a tornado watch and warning—What needs to be done? Who should do what job? Where will you go? Hold family tornado drills so everyone knows what to do and where to go. Encourage children to ask questions and participate in the discussion.

Devastating Hurricanes

Note: If hurricanes do not occur in the area where you live, you may want to skip this section with your class.

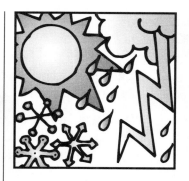

The Rules	The Reasons
Learn the meaning of a hurricane watch and a hurricane warning.	A hurricane **watch** means a hurricane may hit land, but not right away. You have time to take precautions. Keep tuned to the radio or television for updated information.
Go to a safe place.	A hurricane **warning** means a hurricane is likely to make landfall within the next 24 hours.
Be prepared.	People who live in low areas may need to seek shelter in a safer place on higher ground.

If your family plans to stay home during a hurricane, they should:

- Tape and board-up windows.
- Check the first-aid kit.
- Get food and water ready.
- Gather waterproof matches, a lantern, and batteries for the radio and flashlights.
- Fill bathtubs and sinks with water.
- Remove all loose objects from the yard, like lawn furniture and bicycles.
- Bring pets inside.
- Leave one or two windows slightly open on the side of the house away from the wind.
- Keep tuned to the radio for emergency broadcasts. Follow the instructions of local authorities.

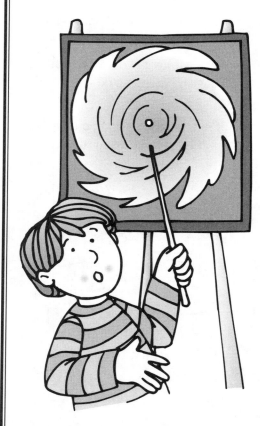

Stay away from windows.	Broken glass can cut you.
Stay inside until the hurricane has passed.	Never go outside during a hurricane. The strong winds are dangerous. Flying objects and broken glass can injure people. Power lines may be broken. Huge waves can cause floods.

Introduction

Hurricanes are major storms with sustained winds of over 75 miles per hour. In the Atlantic and eastern Pacific region, the storms are called hurricanes. The word *hurricane* comes from the West Indian word *huracan*, meaning "big wind." In the western Pacific, these storms are known as typhoons, from the Chinese word *taifun*, meaning "great wind."

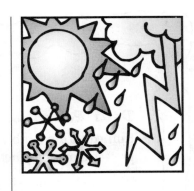

The center of a hurricane contains an "eye," a cloud-free circular region with relatively light winds, six to sixty miles wide. Around the eye, winds rotate counter-clockwise at extremely high speeds.

Damage from hurricanes is caused not only by high winds, but also by flooding due to torrential rains, high waves, and tides.

Hurricane intensity is measured from one to five on the Saffur-Simpson scale. The scale is used to estimate the potential property damage and flooding expected along the coast from a hurricane landfall. Wind speed is the determining factor in the scale. Storm surge is the number of feet above normal tides.

Category	Wind Speed	Severity	Storm Surge
1	74–95 MPH	Weak	4–5 feet
2	96–110 MPH	Moderate	6–8 feet
3	111–130 MPH	Strong	9–12 feet
4	131–155 MPH	Very Strong	13–18 feet
5	155+ MPH	Devastating	18+ feet

Luckily, hurricanes can be tracked by radar via satellite, giving meteorologists clear pictures of the size and intensity of a hurricane long before it reaches land. This ability to watch hurricanes develop and track their speed and direction, has enabled meteorologists to issue warnings well in advance of landfall.

We cannot stop the terrible destruction of hurricanes, but people can be much safer by following hurricane-safety guidelines.

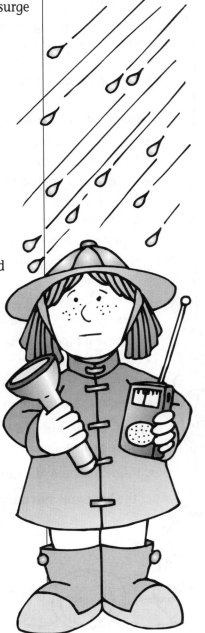

Discussion

Have you ever been in a hurricane? What was it like? If a hurricane was coming and you had to leave your home for a few days, what would you pack if you could only take one suitcase?

Activity

If hurricanes occur in your area, invite someone from the local emergency government or appropriate organization to speak about what to do during a hurricane watch and warning. Encourage children to ask questions and participate in the discussion.

Dear Parents,

Hurricanes are terrible storms that can cause much damage to property and injure people who are not protected and prepared. Most hurricanes occur between June and December.

We have been studying about hurricane safety in class. Please review the hurricane-safety guidelines with your family. We cannot stop the terrible destruction of a hurricane, but people can be much safer by following hurricane-safety guidelines and by getting out of its path.

When a hurricane **watch** is issued, it means a hurricane may hit land, but not right away. You have time to take precautions. Keep tuned to the radio for updated information and double-check your preparations.

A hurricane **warning** means a hurricane is likely to occur within the next 24 hours. Finalize preparations for leaving the area if it becomes necessary. People who live in low areas may need to seek shelter in a safer place on higher ground, 15 to 20 miles away from the coast. Determine a quick, dependable route to a safer place. Have the car gassed, packed, and ready to go.

If you plan to stay home during a hurricane:

- Tape and board-up windows.
- Prepare a fully-stocked first-aid kit with a first-aid manual.
- Have tools available to quickly shut off gas and water heaters.
- Prepare a stock of canned goods, dried foods, powdered milk, and water. Plan enough food and water for your family for at least three days.
- A camping stove can be used for outdoor cooking in case the gas and electricity are out.
- Make certain you have waterproof matches, a lantern, and batteries for the radio and flashlights.
- Fill bathtubs and sinks with water.
- Turn the refrigerator to the coldest setting. Open it as little as possible.
- Remove all loose objects from the yard, like lawn furniture and bicycles.
- Bring pets inside.
- Leave one or two windows slightly open on the side of the house away from the wind.
- Keep tuned to the radio for emergency broadcasts. Follow instructions of local authorities.

Never go outside during a hurricane. The strong winds are dangerous. Flying objects and broken glass can injure people. Power lines may be broken. Huge waves can cause floods.

Stay inside until the hurricane has passed. Stay away from windows.

After the hurricane has passed, watch out for downed power lines.

Unpredictable Earthquakes

Note: If earthquakes do not occur in the area where you live, you may wish to skip this section with your class.

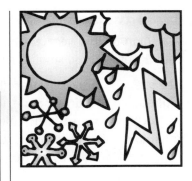

The Rules	The Reasons
Since earthquakes cannot be predicted, know what to do ahead of time if an eqrthquake occurs.	Talk to your parents about what to do if you are at home, at school, shopping, or at a friend's house.

During an Earthquake:

The Rules	The Reasons
If you are indoors when an earthquake happens, stay there. Get under a heavy table, desk, or bed. Cover your head with a pillow, book, or magazine.	Heavy furniture can protect you from falling objects.
Stay away from windows and mirrors.	You could be cut by broken glass if they break.
If you are in a high building, stay out of the elevators and stairways.	If the power goes out, the elevators will not work. Stairs can collapse during an earthquake.
If you are outside, move away from high buildings, walls, power poles, or other tall objects. Move to an open area if possible.	Earthquakes can cause buildings to collapse and objects to fall.
Watch out for downed power lines.	Broken power lines or lines on the ground could cause electrical shock.
Remain calm.	Earthquakes are scary. Remember the rules above to be as safe as possible.

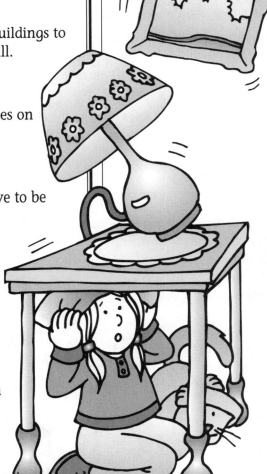

After an Earthquake:

The Rules	The Reasons
Don't use telephones except in an emergency.	Keep the lines open for emergency calls.
Do not light matches or turn on lights.	This may cause a fire or explosion if there are any gas leaks.
Be aware of water contamination. Do not drink, wash food in, or bathe in contaminated water.	Contaminated water can make you very sick.

Introduction

A million times a year, earthquakes occur someplace in the world. Most earthquakes are minor. Some are so small they are not even felt.

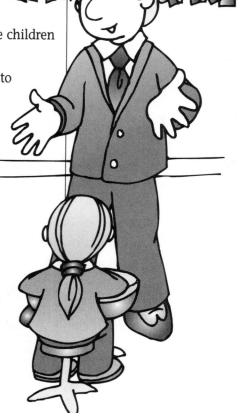

The strength of the seismic sound waves emitted by an earthquake is measured on a scale called the Richter scale, named for seismologist Charles Richter. The scale, from 1 to 10, includes one-tenth increments. A difference of one whole number on the scale reflects a ten-fold factor of earthquake intensity. Earthquakes that measure 6.0 or more are considered dangerous. In North America, the most powerful earthquake recorded was 8.5 in Alaska in 1964.

Since it is not possible to predict or issue warnings of an earthquake in advance, everyone who lives in an area where earthquakes occur should be prepared. Children need to discuss with their families what to do during and after an earthquake. They need to know where to go after an earthquake if they are not home when one occurs.

Discussion

Have you ever felt an earthquake? What was it like? What did you do? What can you and your family do to be prepared for an earthquake? What should you do if you are at school during an earthquake?

Activities

Hold earthquake drills. Have children practice the rules on the previous page. Above all, encourage children to remain calm.

Review the procedures in your school for what to do if an earthquake occurs while children are in school. If in school, but not in the classroom, what should they do? Where should they go after the earthquake is over? Where is the designated meeting place for your class?

Invite a seismologist to explain to the class what causes earthquakes. Encourage children to participate in the discussion and ask questions.

Invite someone from the local emergency government department or Red Cross to discuss safety following an earthquake. Encourage children to participate in the discussion.

Send a copy of the parent letter on page 129 home with each child. Encourage children to talk with their parents about what they should do during and after an earthquake.

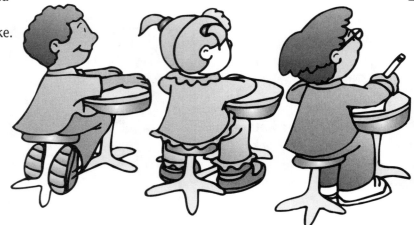

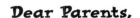

Dear Parents,

We have been discussing earthquake safety in class. A million times a year, earthquakes occur someplace in the world. Most earthquakes are minor. Some are so small they are not even felt.

Since it is not possible to predict earthquakes or issue warnings in advance, everyone who lives in an area where earthquakes occur should be prepared.

Before an Earthquake:

Talk to children about what to do during and after an earthquake. They need to know where to go after an earthquake if they are not home when one occurs.

Have the following items available:

- Fully stocked first-aid kit and first-aid manual
- Canned goods, dried cereal, and powdered milk
- Hand-operated can opener
- Bottled water—at least three gallons per family member per day, plus additional water for pets
- Hand tools, like screwdrivers, pliers, and a hammer
- Camping stove for outside use only
- Portable radios, flashlights, and spare batteries
- Spare set of clothes for each member of the family

Below are the safety rules we discussed in class:

During an Earthquake:

If you are indoors when an earthquake happens, stay there. Get under a heavy table, desk, or bed. Cover your head with a pillow, book, or magazine. Stay away from windows and mirrors.
If you are in a high building, stay out of elevators and stairways.
If you are outside, move away from high buildings, walls, power poles, or other tall objects. Move to an open area if possible.
Remain calm.

After an Earthquake:

Watch out for downed power lines.
Use telephones only in an emergency. Keep the lines open for emergency calls.
Do not light matches or turn on lights. If there are any gas leaks, it may cause a fire or explosion.
Be aware of water contamination. Do not drink, wash food in, or bathe in contaminated water.

S-A-F-E Bingo

Children can review many of the safety rules they've learned while having fun playing S-A-F-E Bingo. Make a copy of pages 130 and 131. Cut apart sentences and place the strips in a box or bag.

Make copies of the S-A-F-E Bingo cards on pages 133–136. You will need one card per child. It will not matter if two children have the same card. Children will need some type of markers or small chips. These can be made from small squares of colored construction paper if you don't have plastic markers.

To Play: Draw one strip of paper and read the sentence to the class. The S, A, F, or E indicates which column children should check. If a child has a picture that matches that sentence, he or she covers that square with a marker. Continue until you have a winner.

To Win: The first child to cover four in a row across, down, or the four corners is the winner. (No diagonals are used in this game.) You can also play "blackout" (all squares must be covered). However, blackout takes longer, and children may get restless.

Small prizes, like pencils, stickers, or hard candy, can be given to the winners.

S • Sara always wears her bike helmet when riding her bicycle.

S • Sam looks both ways before crossing the street.

S • Devan never accepts rides with strangers.

S • Kris always wears a batting helmet when she plays baseball.

S • Trevor always wears a face mask when he is the catcher.

S • Carlos always wears safety equipment when he goes in-line skating.

S • Maria always wears safety equipment when she goes skateboarding.

S • Roberto crosses only at corners or crosswalks.

S • Marsha always waits for the WALK signal before crossing the street.

S • Tomas always dresses warmly when it is cold outside.

A • Gina uses sunscreen when it is hot outside.

A • Kristin never pets or feeds strange animals.

A • Max never plays with matches.

A • Toni keeps both hands on the handlebars when he rides his bike.

A • Jill and Jan always ride their bikes single file.

A • Megan has a smoke detector in her garage.

A • Karl has a fire extinguisher in his kitchen.

Reproducible

S-A-F-E Bingo

A • Brandon builds safe campfires with his dad.

A • Trevor stays on the trail with his friends when hiking.

A • Daisy knows how to Stop! Drop! and Roll!

F • Don knows EXIT signs show the way out.

F • Hal's family stores hazardous products in a locked cabinet.

F • Mark's family has a metal screen in front of the fireplace.

F • Sylvia uses oven mitts to take bowls out of the microwave.

F • Beth's family always remembers to turn pan handles towards the back of the stove.

F • Liz removes cords by pulling on the plug.

F • Stephanie's family has a non-slip mat in the bathtub.

F • Tom picks up his toys so no one will fall over them.

F • Bob puts away tools when he finishes using them.

F • Roberto uses a step stool to reach high shelves.

E • Kisha has a nightlight in her bedroom.

E • Amy takes medicine only when her mom or dad gives it to her.

E • Eun-Jung flies her kite away from trees and power lines.

E • Mike's dad keep his hunting rifle in a locked cabinet.

E • Paula always wears a life jacket at the beach.

E • Rhonda uses the handrails when she goes into the pool.

E • Rick stays seated until the school bus stops.

E • Rachel uses the handrail when she leaves the bus.

E • Renee knows where her family's first-aid kit is kept.

E • Lynn knows how to wash a small cut and put on a bandage.

S-A-F-E BINGO

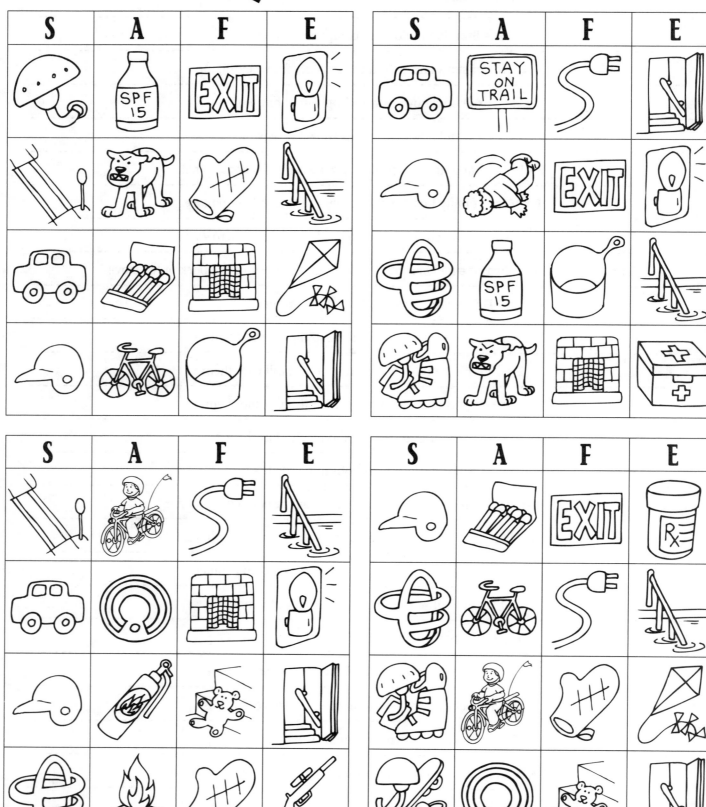

Reproducible © Fearon Teacher Aids FE7959

S-A-F-E Bingo

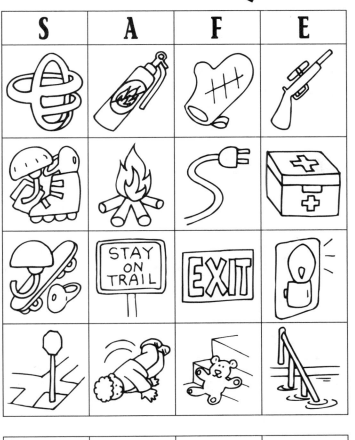

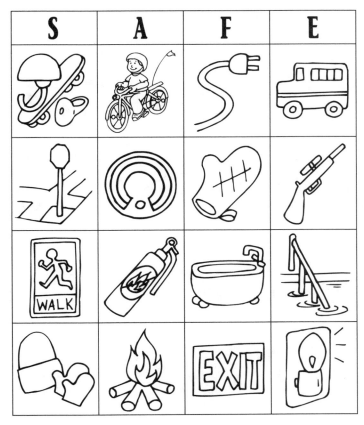

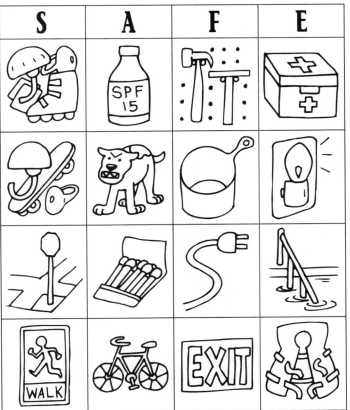

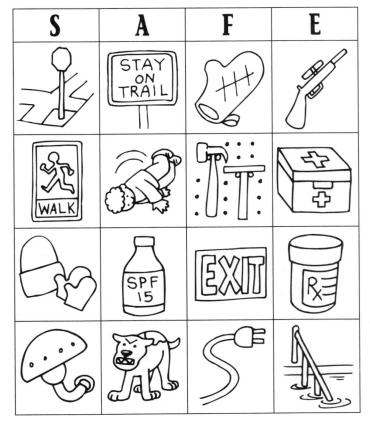

S-A-F-E Bingo

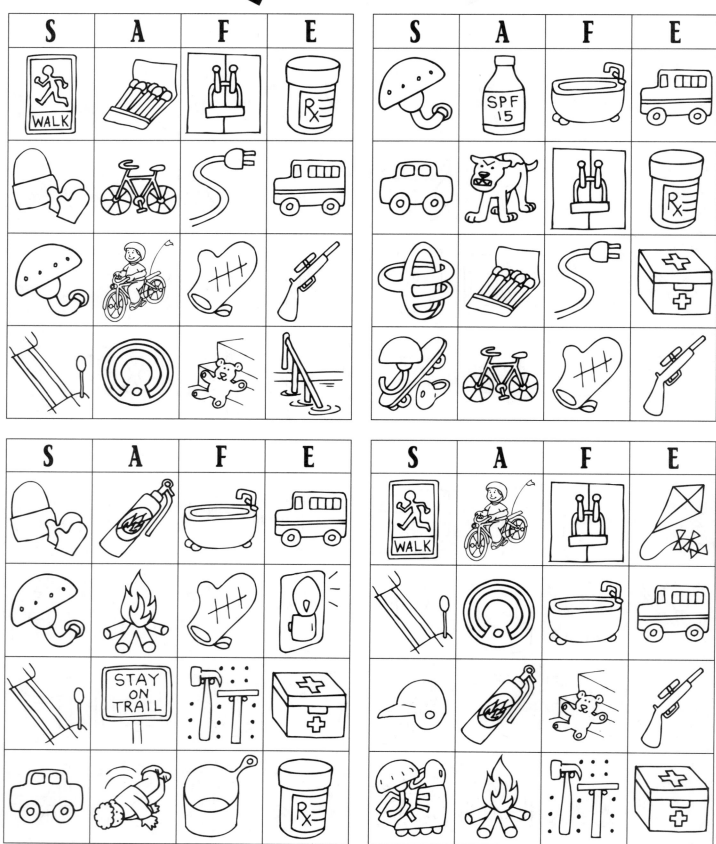

Reproducible

S-A-F-E BINGO

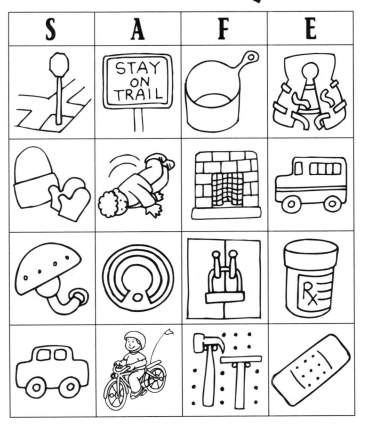

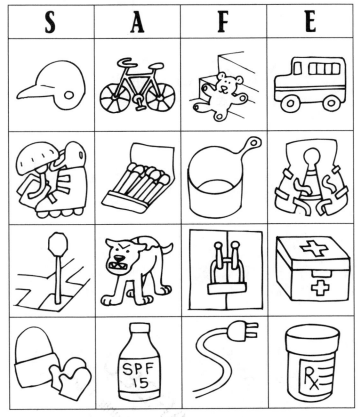

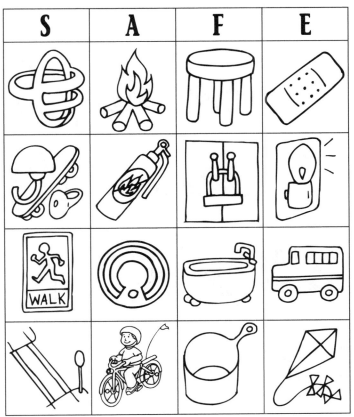

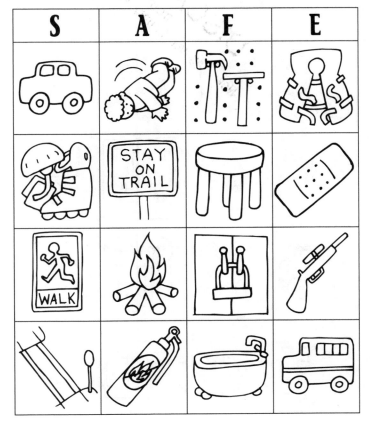

Reproducible

S-A-F-E Bingo

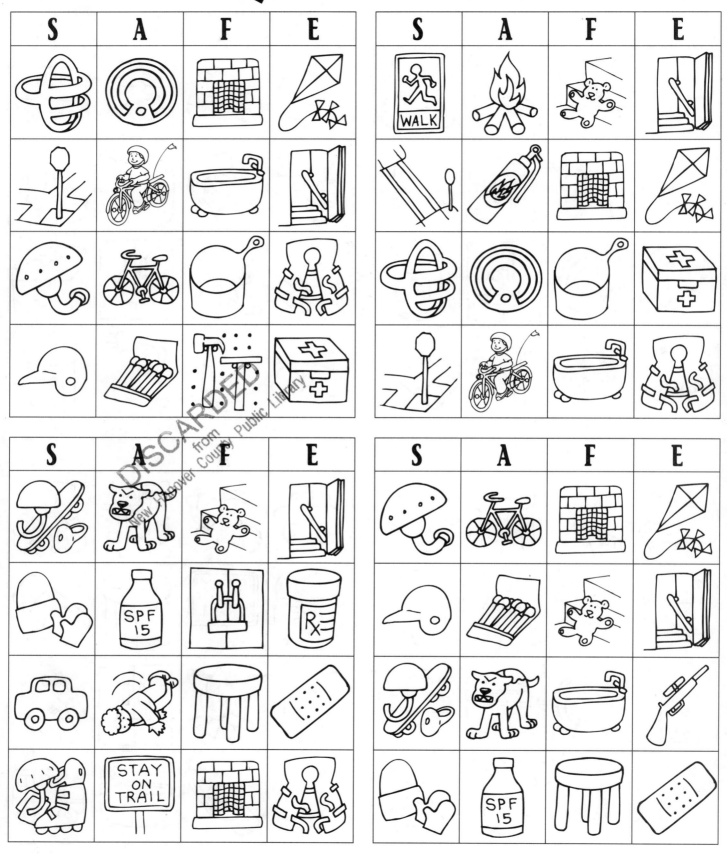

Reproducible